Transform
Your Skin
Naturally

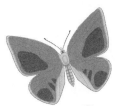

Transform
Your Skin
Naturally

Groundbreaking Alternatives
to Exfoliation and Other
Damaging Antiaging
Strategies

by Ben Johnson, MD

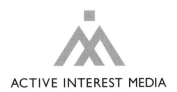

ACTIVE INTEREST MEDIA

Published by:
Active Interest Media, Inc.
300 N. Continental Blvd., Suite 650
El Segundo, CA 90245

Text design by Karen Sperry
Cover design by Silke Design

The information in this book is for educational purposes only and is not recommended as a means of diagnosing or treating an illness. All health matters should be supervised by a qualified healthcare professional. The publisher and the author are not responsible for individuals who choose to self-diagnose and/or self-treat.

Library of Congress Cataloging-in-Publication Data
Johnson, Ben
Transform Your Skin / Ben Johnson
Includes bibliographical references and index.
1. Skin 2. Antiaging 3. Health 4. Integrative Treatment 5. Body Care 6. Title

ISSN: 978-1-935297-35-2

Printed in the United States of America

Acknowledgments

I WANT TO THANK my wife and best friend, Tammy, who has been a source of inspiration and an incredibly patient and supportive partner. I also want to thank my four children, Brandon, Alex, Cassie, and Sophia, for their unconditional love, patience, and understanding through the "crazy" and busy years leading up to this book. Lastly, I would like to thank my editors, Deirdre Shevlin Bell, Matt Plavnick, Lauren Piscopo, and Kim Erickson, for helping me to finally get my thoughts on paper.

Please Note

Contents

Introduction IX

PART 1 STATE OF THE SKIN

Chapter 1 Back to Basics: How Healthy Skin Functions 3

Chapter 2 Skin Care Today: Where We've Gone Astray 19

PART 2 BE GOOD TO YOUR SKIN

Chapter 3 Common Cosmetic Procedures 41

Chapter 4 What's in Your Makeup Bag? A Look at Popular
Ingredients in Cosmetics 59

**PART 3 DR. JOHNSON'S PLAN FOR
YOUTHFUL, HEALTHY SKIN**

Chapter 5 The Basic Plan: Work with the Skin 75

Chapter 6 Healthy Skin from the Inside Out: Nutrition, the
Digestive Tract, and Our Skin 89

Chapter 7 Sun and Sun Protection 107

PART 4 SOLUTIONS FOR PROBLEM SKIN

Chapter 8 Turning Back the Clock 125

Chapter 9 Skin Conditions, Common Approaches,
and Preferred Treatments 141

Conclusion Fixing Problem Skin—For Good 175

APPENDICES

Top 50 Skin Questions Answered 181

Glossary 195

Selected References 203

Index 210

Introduction

~

Even in America, which prides itself
as a society that values innovation,
outmoded ideas persist in how we approach
and treat the skin.

~

IN THE PAST DECADE, much has been written about skincare, with a large focus on choosing the right products. It makes sense that consumers would need guidance, considering the wide variety of options currently on the market today. Skincare treatments range from natural to chemical, organic to medical. It can be hard to navigate the combination of products and treatments, and the subtle degrees of difference often skew the comparisons. Unfortunately, people seeking clarity through published material may find themselves even more confused. It seems that each product is backed by definitive books and articles written to assist the consumer in understanding why Product X is the exact right one for him or her.

Of course, all of these books contain helpful and informative elements, but many simply repeat the same "conventional wisdom" or

~

Our challenge is to understand whether
inflammation is the cause of the problem,
or merely a symptom.

~

dermatological fads and the unproven exfoliation trends that have persisted for decades. The purpose of this book is instead to share ideas that are slightly more outside the box than current therapies and strategies. I will discuss why humans experience the various skin reactions that we do. By understanding what takes place on the skin's surface, and the underlying causes, we can better inform ourselves in order to discover which products and treatments really work to repair and improve the health of the skin.

Global Skin Crisis

I think we can all agree that the state of our skin's health is currently in doubt. Research reports significant increases in skin cancer around the globe., We are also seeing increases in conditions such as rosacea, melasma, eczema, and psoriasis. While I would not put the blame for those conditions solely on our skincare products, I do believe the skincare developments over the last 30 years—which have focused largely on exfoliation, a treatment known to increase inflammation—contribute to the higher incidence of these skin conditions. Clearly, our current model for addressing skin issues is flawed. There is also the visible evidence (amassed from the millions of people who have been trying these inflammation-producing approaches) that undoubtedly shows that what we are doing has not reversed aging or damage.

One of the most interesting things I have found in both my medical research and my own formulating efforts is the human tendency to resist change. Even in America, which prides itself as an innovative society, outmoded ideas persist in how we approach and treat the skin. And never mind how much knowledge and information has been shared and proposed with regard to the various options for treating aging, hyperpigmentation, acne, rosacea, and the many other skin conditions that are common in the United States. At the end of the day, we're still trying the same inflammation-promoting strategies.

The theories utilized by skincare professionals to treat the skin are often flawed, and yet no one seems to be addressing this very basic problem in the skincare industry. That omission is what this book seeks to remedy.

How Did We Get Here?

Before we launch into critical reviews and progressive recommendations on the subject of modern skincare, it's important to understand how skincare treatments have evolved over time. It's also important to understand how products are sold in today's dermatological marketplace. The second consideration is, arguably, more important to us than the first. So even before we explore the history of skincare, let's take a look at the environment in which products and treatments are developed, marketed, and consumed.

Ours is a culture of instant gratification, especially where our health and vanity are concerned. We expect results quickly, if not immediately. All of this is compounded when we part with our hard-earned cash in order to achieve beauty. We want results, and we want them now.

The number one way to make your skin look better in five minutes or in an hour or over the course of a day or two is to actually create more inflammation. Enter a whole class of treatments designed to provide immediate results. Retinoic acid and many retinols, alpha hydroxy acids, lasers, photorejuvenation, excess topical vitamin C, and other therapies provide results by inflaming, peeling, and lightening the skin's uppermost layer. But there is a flaw in these therapies: Instant improvement in appearance results from plumping of the skin, and plumping is almost always caused by localized swelling, or as the result of inflammation. Unfortunately, the vast majority of treatments on the market today are not designed for long-term improvement of the skin because long-term improvement of the skin is usually a slow, meticulous process. The average consumer simply doesn't have the patience for that.

The reason patients and consumers like so many of these modern treatments is because their fine lines look better when the surrounding tissues have been plumped. But plumping is the result of inflammation, and inflammation damages and ages the skin.

I understand the immediate gratification these treatments provide. The problem, however, is that when you inflame the skin daily for temporary results, the long-term consequences actually worsen skin health. For example, applying an alpha hydroxy acid to your face every day increases free-radical exposure (damaging molecules that are missing an electron), as well as increasing the DNA damage that occurs at the cellular level. It also increases the potential for long-term hyperpigmentation and boosts the risk of developing skin cancer. We have long understood that inflammation is the cause of most skin conditions. We also know that alpha hydroxys trigger inflammation in the skin because of their acidic nature. Such acids also damage our protective barrier and increase the amount of sun damage that we accumulate on a daily basis.

The key to understanding any of the commonly used ingredients being marketed is to ask the question, "How does this work on the skin?" The answer for alpha hydroxy acids like glycolic acid is simple: There are no skin receptors that recognize these acids; there is no magical communication that occurs, no physiologic benefit. Sadly, the only way these acids work is by inflaming and destroying our protective barrier.

That said, treatments such as alpha hydroxy acids sell so well precisely because consumers get the results they are looking for, at least in the short term. And no skincare executive in her right mind would attempt to change the status quo, because each of these products requires regular, repeated application. This, in turn requires the user to repeatedly *buy more product*. Add to that the fact that these short-term results lead to long-term negative consequences that will require even more skincare, and skincare companies see only opportunity in the current approach. Most, if not all, skincare companies have product lines to accommodate aging consumers. It's a win-win situation for the skincare industry: Yesterday we sold you a cleansing acne scrub, today we sell you a botanical toning compound, and tomorrow we'll sell you an age-defying cream.

~

Instant improvement in appearance generally results from plumping of the skin. And plumping is often . . . the result of inflammation.

~

It certainly has been a good financial model for these companies over the last few decades. That is not to say that the manufacturers believe they are creating harmful effects; they are just sticking with the current ideology because that is what consumers have been taught to buy.

Understanding the Basics of Skin Conditions

A fundamental premise of my skincare philosophy is that each and every skin condition is caused, at least in part, by inflammation. Let me repeat that: Every single skin condition has an element of inflammation related to it. In itself, this is not big news. However, we have to determine whether that inflammation is local or systemic. In other words, our challenge is to understand whether the inflammation is the cause of the problem, or merely a symptom. Let's take, for example, melasma, a fairly common darkening of the skin that is prevalent among pregnant women and those taking birth-control pills. Is melasma caused by a local disturbance or imbalance, or is it caused by a systemic disturbance or imbalance? The direct relationship to higher or altered hormone levels and melasma should tell us this is a systemically derived condition. Therefore, equal attention should be given to potential internal sources of inflammation, in addition to topical remedies.

This is where we begin to see division among experts. I am situated in the camp with scientists and researchers who believe that internal causes create the vast majority of skin problems. This would include conditions like acne, melasma, psoriasis, eczema, rosacea, and even aging. We have to remember that the American diet is often highly inflammatory, and inflammation is going to change cortisol levels and affect our immune system. All of these factors will impact an individual's ability to heal and to manage specific skin disturbances.

Reconsidering Skin Conditions

Consider acne for a moment. Countless people of all ages experience acne every year, and it is theorized that about a third of these cases are related to an internal yeast overgrowth within the system, often in the colon. My own anecdotal research supports this theory. Hormone levels also contribute to acne. This is why people with excessive testosterone levels tend to suffer from it, as do women during menstruation. In addition, immune-challenged individuals who often, through poor dietary choices, create an internal environment that promotes the overgrowth of bacteria on the skin, often suffer from acne.

Typical approaches to acne include topical regimens, as well as internal regimens like antibiotics, spironolactone, Accutane, or birth control pills. All of these options are going to be discussed in the coming chapters, but none of them address why these physiologic changes occur. They also don't provide solutions to eradicate excess yeast or offer dietary management strategies to allow the immune system to combat bacterial overgrowth.

We can also discuss the same issues as they relate to psoriasis. There is clearly an internal cause for psoriasis, which explains the waxing and waning of skin irritation. The only prescription-based psoriasis therapies currently being offered are topical drugs and/or internal drugs that suppress the immune system—as if it is the immune system's fault that it is out of control. Again it would be my opinion that it is not the immune system that is out of control; instead, I believe we can find an underlying cause that leads to such a chronic skin problem.

The same thing is true of rosacea. I am a firm believer that rosacea is primarily a digestive tract issue that shows itself on the skin. The fact that there is a huge increase in rosacea sufferers in the United States suggests that we need to seriously address the dietary habits of this country. That's a generalization, though, and hardly a pointed solution or set of steps that the rosacea sufferer might follow for relief. When we take skin complaints on a case-by-case basis, however, it becomes easy to provide guidance—which we will do in this book—to better manage these conditions from multiple points of view.

~

All these acids, chemicals, and treatments such as
lasers and intense light therapy focus on making
the skin look healthier. This is not the
same as actually *creating* healthier skin.

~

Understanding What Current Therapies Actually Do

To truly appreciate the development of skincare treatments throughout human history, and to really understand how bankrupt our current
approach is, we should discuss what our popular therapies actually do to
the skin and why we choose to believe that the results are desirable. We've
already noted that the modern cure to wrinkles and fine lines is to induce
swelling in the tissues around the target area. (I use the term *swelling* in
place of the word *plumping* to reinforce the notion that our actions and
therapies actually insult the skin. Swelling is a healing reaction provoked
by injury; let's remember that so much of modern dermatological treatment is based on the concept of doing harm.) What we fail to appreciate,
however, is the long-term effect such treatment has on the skin.

For a better sense of the long-term effects of popular skin treatments,
let's break down the processes involved in treating skin conditions with
alpha hydroxy acids, which is a very common approach today. To begin,
let's clarify that alpha hydroxy acids include glycolic acid, lactic acid,
malic acid, citric acid, and tartaric acid. Each of these, in turn, is naturally
occurring and can be derived from (in order mentioned) sugar cane,
milk, apples, citrus fruits, and grapes. These substances have been used
for skincare for centuries. Cleopatra famously used baths of milk and
rose petals to exfoliate and nourish her skin. What may confuse many
consumers who assume that naturally derived ingredients are good for
the body and skin is that there is little, if any, healthy effect created by
using these acids. There are no receptors in the skin that these acids communicate with so the only message they can send is one of "fix this!"

resulting from the blunt trauma they inflict. In addition, even though it sounds nice that these acids can be extracted from fruit, they never are. The cosmetics industry only uses synthetically derived acids because natural sources are typically too expensive.

Glycolic acid makes an interesting study to help us understand the landscape of today's treatments. Glycolic acid is the chief agent in most chemical peels performed at spas or skincare clinics and in kits for at-home use. The smallest of all alpha hydroxy acids (molecularly), glycolic acid melts through the surface layer of skin, removing our protective lipids and surface skin cells in the process. This immediately leads to an inflammatory response and skin plumping—which is why it is still popular. The downside is that we have triggered inflammation, an aging event in itself. This single application sets the skin up to age significantly more quickly over the next few days. How? The removal of our protective barrier allows for more ultraviolet (UV) damage until the skin can repair itself. There is also a greater demand for the essential nutrients that help to restore skin tissue. As a result, these nutrients can be depleted, leaving the skin in short supply. It also reduces the amount of melanin in your skin, leading to even more free-radical damage. None of this accounts for the challenges the initial inflammation created. Bottom line? Nothing good comes from the application of glycolic acid.

Of course, we should remember that glycolic acid is an acid. Its effect, mild as it may be, is to corrode and eliminate the outer surface of the skin. When we consider its application in terms of a chemical peel, the dangers increase. Now the intent is not just to slough dead skin and increase epidermal turnover, it is to seriously maim the skin so that it is forced to replace the entire barrier. Doesn't the whole concept sound a little barbaric? Also remember that forcing your skin to replace the epidermis, while it seems rejuvenating, is not really an anti-aging activity since the epidermis is not the layer of your skin where wrinkles are born.

I understand the immediate gratification involved in such a treatment, both for the client and the provider. First, alpha hydroxy acids can be relatively inexpensive and easy to use at home to achieve the desired

Cleopatra's renowned skincare secret worked
because the lactic acid in that legendary
milk bath gently removes dead skin cells
while also hydrating the skin.

results. And if you're going to spend anywhere from $100 to $500 at a spa or with a skincare specialist, you want to see results immediately.

The flaw in this strategy is that all of these acids, chemicals, and treatments such as lasers and intense light therapy focus on making the skin *look* healthier. This is not the same as actually *creating* healthier skin. Developing healthier skin takes much more time and effort, and it involves changes inside the body, which we'll address in later chapters. Alas, such change is much harder to market and sell. And as long as customers are happy with the results of a chemical peel or a laser treatment, then I suspect the skincare industry will not rush to change the status quo.

The Problem with Current Skincare Solutions

If customers are happy, and if skincare professionals continue to use technology to find new ways to affect the same results, namely the removal of dead skin cells, then is it really such a bad practice? Exfoliation is so common that it's become standard fare at most spas in America and part of many at-home skin regimens. If it weren't good for us, would we still be doing it?

As we've discussed, the vast majority of procedures on the market today are not designed for long-term improvement of the skin. Long-term improvement is a slower, more meticulous process, and, to be blunt, consumers generally don't have the patience for it. That is not to say that alternative treatments discussed later in the book are not immediately noticeable, because they often are; it is just that inflammatory products create a more extreme response. Consumers look for treatments that create an instant improvement in wrinkles and blemishes.

~

Of course, we should remember that
glycolic acid is *acid*. When we consider
the chemical peel in these terms,
it's much harder to escape the reality that
glycolic acid is *burning* the skin.

~

And the most common way to achieve this improvement is to incite plumping, and this almost universally involves inflammation. Also, these treatments don't last, and reapplication and repetition are requisite to maintaining the desired appearance—which again makes the point that these are *temporary* results.

The flaw here is that, when you incite inflammation, the long-term consequences result in more rapid aging. The skin is obviously worse off as a result of this daily barrage of inflammation. The skin already thins at an average of about 1 percent per year at the dermal level (the layer of skin just below the epidermis, consisting of blood vessels and connective tissue). Adding inflammation to the natural thinning process is a recipe for further deterioration. It results in more DNA damage, loss of stem cells, the rapid evolution of uneven skin tone and age spots, higher risk of skin cancer, and a host of cellular issues that continue to compromise the health of the skin. Given these considerations, inflaming the skin even further can't possibly lead to long-term improvements. Even if trauma does cause an increase in collagen production, there is still a lingering question: Does that increased collagen get applied to old or new damage? The answer is obviously the latter. If a burn results in a spike of collagen production, it would only make sense that the collagen is being made to repair the burn. We rely on modern approaches to interrupt the skin's natural function and we never allow the skin to restore its own balance.

At this point, it is fair to suggest that 30 years of anecdotal evidence and research from around the world supports that we have not been making our skin younger or healthier. Retin-A®, glycolic acid, and the barrage of traumatic laser and related treatments are not creating long-term benefits. If any of these treatments was truly rebuilding the skin, we would all use it to help us look like we were 25 again.

Once you get past the question of whether or not skin conditions come from internal causes, we have to identify options for treating those skin conditions. This again is where a philosophical divide separates practitioners. I am of the opinion that the approach to these skin conditions needs to be holistic. I use the word *holistic* not to suggest solutions must be organic, all-natural, or full of, as I call them, "froufrou ingredients" that gently caress and moisturize the skin. I do not actually believe that expensive lotions and razzle-dazzle botanicals by themselves are an effective strategy for anyone.

Most of the treatments that are currently prescribed and/or recommended by skincare professionals either promote inflammation or they result in immunosuppression of the normal functions of skin remodeling and repair, both of which are detrimental. My position is based on a couple of key points. First, the skin is a remarkable and wondrous organ. The more research that is done, the more we realize that all of the skin's different functions and responses to physiologic imbalances

Dermatitis

The word *dermatitis* literally means "inflammation of the skin." As we explore various skincare attitudes, products, and treatments, it's important to remember that all of the skin conditions we discuss in this book are forms of dermatitis. When a dermatologist prescribes a cream or steroid, he's looking to interrupt or suppress an inflammation in the skin.

When you have an adverse skin reaction, your skin is adjusting to chemical or physical imbalances and is trying to compensate for those imbalances. Too many skin professionals are prone to *interrupting* the skin's reactions. As you'll see throughout this book, my approach is to work *with* the skin's reaction and identify ways to restore balance rather than simply suppress inflammation.

Skin Remodeling

You will encounter the term *skin remodeling* throughout this book, and it's important to understand what it means. Skin remodeling is the process by which our body removes damaged skin cells and replaces them with normal, healthy ones. As children, the process of skin remodeling is fast and flawless, but the process slows dramatically as we age. This means slower wound healing, longer-lasting blemishes, and greater impact from environmental assaults like sun damage. My approach to skincare is based on the idea that we can restore and maintain our skin's remodeling abilities as we age. The end result: diminished wrinkles, reduced sun damage, and overall healthy, youthful skin.

are so complex and so phenomenally accurate that it is arrogant for skincare professionals to think that we know better than the skin. The primary focus of any remedy or topical cream should be to *assist* the skin in healing the condition, as opposed to interfering with normal physiologic activity. Unfortunately, we too often see skincare professionals attempting to treat the symptoms rather than addressing the underlying causes.

I think the vast majority of researchers working on skincare products today believe that outbreaks are the result of the skin behaving abnormally. Take psoriasis, for example. Many professionals believe that psoriasis is the result of skin that is behaving erratically and out of control. Too many practitioners assume that the skin is not aware of itself or that the skin can't control its own dysfunction. From this perspective, it's easy to understand why so many physicians and skincare professionals assume it is their role to interfere with the skin's normal activity in order to achieve a result. This is a standard protocol for many physicians who, in good faith, offer steroid creams to improve symptoms.

Of course, this approach provides relief from symptoms, and for the most part, that is why people visit dermatologists. However, this

*Before we invest another dollar in improving
our skin from the outside in, we must
look long and hard at whether
the cost of today's radiance is worth
more aggravation tomorrow.*

approach does not address the internal imbalance that led to the condition in the first place. If we only treat the symptoms, then we often can only offer temporary skincare solutions.

As you will read in the chapters forthcoming, we can address and identify many of these internal imbalances, thereby better managing these skin conditions from a combined approach of restoring skin health without interfering with the normal physiological processes of the skin. In addition, we can address and stabilize the underlying condition. In this way, skincare professionals and clients can work together to achieve long-term skin health.

Turning Point

In the 1970s, scientists unveiled the "antiaging" properties of tretinoin, the acid form of vitamin A. Tretinoin, commonly known today as Retin-A®, has enjoyed wild popularity because it is touted as an effective way to treat acne and restore the appearance of youthfulness to the skin. With the earlier discovery and application of many of the chemicals we've discussed, and with advances in light technology such as lasers and photorejuvenation treatments, the marketing of skincare products has taken on a whole new dimension during the past three decades. Over the past 30 years, the emphasis has turned to restoring the skin's youth and vitality based on processes that likely *accelerate* aging.

One way to reverse the trend of damaging the skin in the name of beauty—an outside-in approach—is to look long and hard at adopting a more holistic approach to skin health. We must recognize that disturbances of the skin reflect imbalances in the whole body. We've long

~

The skin is a remarkable and
wondrous organ.

~

known that diet and lifestyle play critical roles in the skin's health. But the corporate skincare industry, as much as it may embrace the use of natural products, is not looking to sell balance and inner harmony as winning skincare ingredients.

Natural skincare approaches go beyond using natural or organic ingredients in lotions, creams, and treatments. As I will discuss later in this book, truly natural skincare borrows from holistic and ancient healing practices, balancing the body's basic systems and elements to achieve more complete skin health. To treat an eruption of the skin is to treat the symptom without addressing the underlying problem. This is the failure of modern dermatology. We must consciously recognize that the trend in all of the current skincare treatments—from penetrating lotions to acid peels to laser surgeries—fails to address the real problem. For all the technology, skincare professionals often insist on treating the symptom without regard for the problem. This will only result in temporary success and long-term failure.

Today we are at a crossroads over 4,000 years in the making. We can continue to assault our skin with harsh treatments that promote inflammation or we can embrace whole-body approach that supports healthy skin inside and out. If we chose the latter, clients, patients, and consumers will all be happier, healthier, and more radiant.

The Bottom Line

The skincare industry has come a long way in the past 50 years, and not always for the better. Today's most popular treatments focus on technology, expedience, and immediate results, much to the detriment of our skin. This trend is based in large part on the workings of our marketplace, on corporate strategy, and on consumer demand.

Today's leading skin treatments introduce inflammation to plump the skin, which reduces the appearance of wrinkles, blemishes, and fine lines. These treatments require repetitive use and reapplication, and our skin actually ages faster as a result. Alpha hydroxy acids, retinoic acid, lasers, and heat-based treatments all come highly recommended, yet all of them come at a cost. For the skincare industry, the cycle of damaged skin is a perfect business plan.

Truly healthful skin starts from the inside out, and very few products can match the skin effects from a strong constitution. Our skin is an integral component—the largest organ in the body! It is a system that is designed to react and regulate in healthful ways, if we let it. Modern skincare approaches fall into the trap of treating symptoms without ever identifying and treating problems. By helping skin achieve balance with the body's basic systems and elements, we can attain results that truly improve the health of our skin.

Whether you are a physician seeking to get beyond traditional medical approaches to skincare; an aesthetician searching out philosophies, methods, and treatments that better resolve your clients' needs; or a layperson looking for skincare answers that, thus far, have eluded you, I hope you'll find this book meets your needs. The bottom line is that toxins, nutritional deficiencies, ineffective skincare practices, and UV exposure present the skin with a set of challenges that require our active participation, working together, to reduce inflammation and promote healing within the skin. This book will help you better understand the most appropriate responses, both topically and holistically, to your dermatological complaints and restore your skin to its optimal functioning.

What's in the Book

It is important for everyone to appreciate the complex nature of skin physiology. In these pages, we'll take a step back so we can understand that the body is designed to adapt. When we eat toxic foods, are exposed to a toxic chemical, or experience imbalance in the body, several adaptations occur to try to maintain good health.

The skin makes every effort to restore itself to a full dermal density as it ages. It does not create acne cysts or an eczema flareup because it is out of control. Precisely the opposite. As you'll see throughout this book, an outbreak is the skin's attempt to control a localized problem that occurs as the result of an internal condition. This is why skincare professionals should work with the body's responses—not against those responses—in an effort to correct the symptoms.

I approached this book from the standpoint that all the efforts we apply to the skin should work in concert with the normal functions of the skin. Yet, too often we assume the skin is incapable of managing itself, and so we interfere with immune function or some other aspect of skin physiology.

One thing you'll discover as you read through these pages is that the deeper we delve into these skin conditions, the more we realize that the skin is a reflection of what is going on inside of us. Unfortunately, by its very nature, the skin often takes the brunt of our bad habits and environmental assaults. In other words, when we smoke or eat toxic foods, there is clearly an effect on the skin's ability to heal and manage inflammation. Combine that with the fact that many of us lack the nutritional support needed to create collagen, fight infection, or heal wounds. This prevents our skin from performing optimally.

Finally, we will get to the most plaguing problem when it comes to skin aesthetics: UV damage. Taken together, these factors—toxins, nutritional deficiencies, and UV exposure—create quite a challenge for this remarkably resilient organ.

This book is, in a sense, written to pay homage to the skin. At the same time, I hope it will help guide all of us in our efforts to control dermatological conditions without abusing the skin. We have to remember that inflammation is a critical component of every skin condition. Unfortunately, over the last few decades, the focus and the intent of the vast majority of procedures and skincare regimens has been to incite inflammation in the name of "treatment." You'll learn more about this as we discuss flawed strategies in skin treatment today.

This leads me to my final point: As a general rule, anything that promotes inflammation should be avoided, because that will only exacerbate whatever skin condition you are already suffering from. It interferes with normal skin health, increases the risk of skin cancer, and leads to more rapid aging as we move into our later years. But, by learning to prevent inflammation and to support your skin's intrinsic healing capacity, you can achieve and maintain healthy, youthful skin for many years to come.

Part 1

~

State of the Skin

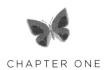

CHAPTER ONE

Back to Basics: How Healthy Skin Functions

BY NOW IT SHOULD come as no surprise that I'm in constant awe and appreciation of how intelligent the skin is. From the time we are in the womb until our last breath, our skin is in a constant state of renewal and repair, 24 hours a day, 7 days a week. While there is certainly a part of our skin health that requires proper nutrition, including certain amino acids and vitamin C, the vast majority of skin function operates semi-independently in a remarkable fashion to maintain itself—no matter what the environment.

In its prime—during childhood and young adulthood—skin performs all its functions to protect the body from environmental harm. It is able to better handle the amount of sun exposure, debris, environmental toxins, and bacteria that it encounters every day. This is the state of skin health that we strive to maintain as we age. But unfortunately, most people experience significant changes in their skin as they get older, and the normal functions that we take for granted become less effective or less efficient. To understand why that happens—and how we can return to an optimal state of skin health—it's important to have some basic knowledge of how our skin works.

Basics of Skin Anatomy

The skin consists of three primary layers: the epidermis (the outer layer), the dermis (the middle layer), and the subcutis (the deepest layer). Let's start with a simple understanding of our epidermis.

EPIDERMIS. The epidermis is the outermost layer of our skin. The fact that the epidermis does not have its own blood supply might seem like a design flaw, but it's simply another piece of evidence of the skin's intelligent design. If we did have capillaries in our epidermis, we would constantly be bleeding every time we bumped into something. Instead, the epidermis forms a protective barrier on the surface of the skin.

Below the epidermis is our dermis. This is the source of our skin's nutrition, most immune/repair activity, and the rightful target for aging (and most other skin-condition) treatments and topicals. Almost everything that the epidermis needs—including vitamins, antioxidants, lipids, amino acids, and other nutrients—comes from the dermis and its abundant blood flow. Every day of our lives, our skin spends a great deal of effort developing the cells that make up the epidermis through a constant nutrient uptake from the dermal food supply. That nutrient uptake is completely dependent on healthy circulation and the efficiency of the skin's cells. These dermal cells include fibroblasts and macrophages, which you'll learn more about in the next section. Oxygen must also be delivered via the blood vessels in the dermis.

The nutrients travel from the dermis to the epidermis through the basal membrane, at the bottom of the epidermis. Sitting upon the basal membrane are a few key cells:

- Keratinocytes make up the bulk of the cells within the epidermis. They sit at the bottom of the epidermis, gathering enough lipids, proteins, and enzymes to be able to mature and develop into the various layers of our protective barrier. The final phase of that development is what is considered to be the "dead" part of our skin, the stratum corneum. Many people blame the "dead skin cells" at the very surface of their skin for wrinkles, uneven skin tone, and dull, lifeless skin—but those cells have nothing to do with it. We need to start respecting how important those cells are in preventing all of

The epidermis is divided primarily into four layers:

- The **basal layer** is the deepest layer of the epidermis. Think of the basal layer as the soil. It is closest to the dermis and it is the conduit for all the nutrients and oxygen the epidermis needs.
- Next is the **stratum spinosum**. Also known as the "spinous" or "prickle-cell" layer, the stratum spinosum has cells that produce lipids that prevent evaporation. This is also the layer in which the production of keratin begins.
- Above the stratum spinosum is the **stratum granulosum**, or granular layer, where keratin proteins and waterproofing lipids are produced and organized.
- The outermost layer of the epidermis is the **stratum corneum**, which is often—and unfortunately—considered the "dead" part of the skin. In fact, it is an essential part of our epidermal barrier and is as an important part of proper skin health.

these skin issues. Those cells are critical in preventing aging, infection, and dehydration, and therefore should not be forced off with exfoliants and peels.

- Lipids are not independent cells within the epidermis, but I list them here because they play such an important role in protecting us from aging and dryness. Lipids act as the primary structure of our cell walls but they are also part of the glue that holds the epidermis together. When there is a shortage or when they are stripped by treatments or chemicals, the skin ages faster and dries out. In addition, the skin allows more environmental toxins in and begins to develop enlarged pores and sebum overproduction.

- Melanocytes produce melanin, or pigment. This type of cell is one of the most important parts of the antiaging story. Melanin is remarkably effective at minimizing the damage from excessive UV exposure and allows us go out in the sun without significant trauma. While we all have similar numbers of melanocytes, they are genetically programmed to produce a specific amount of melanin at rest and a maximum amount of melanin in the presence of sun damage. People with darker skin obviously have an advantage, which is why they may not start wrinkling as soon as Caucasians with lighter skin.

- Stem cells are getting a lot of attention for their potential in several aspects of aging. They also have great potential in skincare. They can provide a source of growth factors and other cell nutrients when their growth media is used topically. More important, however, is the nurturing of the stem cells that are naturally housed in the epidermis and dermis. This is an important part of my approach.

Even though our dermis is our most important target for skincare strategies, the skin actually gives priority to the epidermis. Our dermis begins thinning between the ages of 20 and 30, and thins approximately 1 percent a year for the rest of our lives. If the epidermis, which experiences marginal thinning, were to thin at 1 percent a year starting at age 20, many of us would likely succumb to death through fluid loss or infection at some point in our 40s. That's because the epidermis prevents overwhelming infections from growing on the skin through its low pH

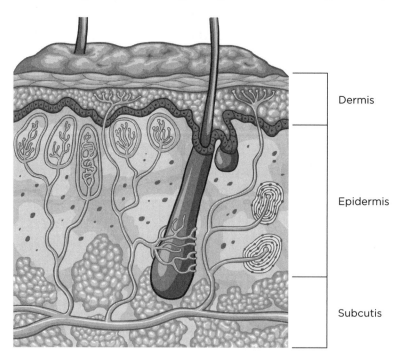

Dermis

Epidermis

Subcutis

stratum corneum function. It also prevents fluid and blood loss through its protective-barrier functions.

For this reason, the skin actually puts a priority on delivering nutrients to the epidermis to make sure it is always intact. Even as we see a reduction in capillary delivery of the skin's nutrition as we age, the epidermis manages to maintain itself by slowing its turnover rate. Unfortunately, this epidermal priority can result in losses to the dermis, which is allowed to thin as we age. The loss of dermal thickness increases wrinkles and sagging but, since dermal thinning does not threaten our health, it has a low likelihood of actually impacting our survival.

The basal (bottom) layer of the epidermis acts like "fertile soil" for the many cells of the epidermis and therefore takes priority. The reason it's such an important part of the skin is because it is the feeding center for our epidermal stem cells, keratinocytes, and melanocytes. Melanocytes need tyrosine, cysteine, copper, and other nutrients in order to maintain adequate pigment production. Keratinocytes need a whole variety of growth factors and cofactors like zinc, copper, and selenium. The dermis must deliver these along with antioxidants, lipids, enzymes, and proteins to continue to repair and maintain the epidermal barrier throughout the entire span of our lives. The skin never has an opportunity to go dormant; it must always continue to function or else we will perish.

As the keratinocyte matures it becomes a corneocyte, which forms the top barrier of our skin in the stratum corneum. This top layer of our skin gets a bad rap: Many skincare professionals believe that since the skin cells are "dead," they're unneeded. That's the basis of the arguments in favor of exfoliation and other procedures that remove "dead skin." The fact is that the stratum corneum is an essential part of a very carefully designed system; it is highly protective of and beneficial to the skin. Its low pH (acidic) environment keeps bacteria from overwhelming the skin and developing into an infection. It is also an area where we have a lipid matrix. This helps prevent water from leaving the skin, and environmental toxins from entering. In addition, the stratum corneum plays a critical role in reflecting 80 percent of damaging UV radiation. When we exfoliate, a lot more UV damage occurs. Remember, your skin exfoliates every day on its own time, when it is ready. When I discuss exfoliation, I am referring to forced exfoliation, in which we are deciding when these protective layers need to be removed. The combination of beneficial functions makes the stratum corneum a crucial component of skin health—and yet, the skincare industry continues to promote exfoliation, dermabrasion, and other aggressive inflammatory procedures that compromise its protective capacity.

As you can see, the epidermis is a complex and valuable part of the skin. Equally important is the layer that provides the epidermis with all its nutrients: the dermis.

DERMIS. The thickest of the three layers of the skin is the dermis, which consists most significantly of collagen, elastin, and glycosaminoglycans (GAGs). Within in the dermal layer, two of the most important cells are the fibroblasts and the macrophages. Let's learn a little about each.

- **Fibroblasts** are the most important cells found in our dermis because they manufacture collagen, elastin, and GAGs. The brilliant function of fibroblasts—and their strategic location—is another bit of proof that the skin is designed intelligently. The skin needs immediate,

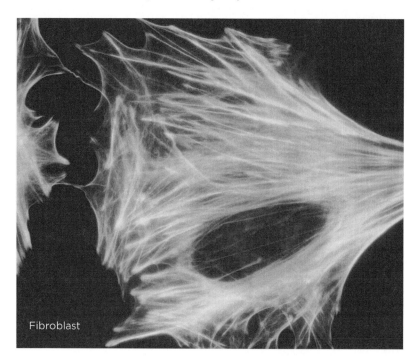

Fibroblast

direct access to nutrient delivery from the capillary beds, so it makes sense that fibroblasts would in fact migrate and maintain themselves in an environment that has a significant amount of circulation and nutrient delivery. Also, because of their vital role, these cells are found in the dermis and not the epidermis, where they would be damaged too significantly by UV rays to maintain themselves as well as they do throughout our lives. Fibroblasts are dependent on several nutrients in order to be healthy and successful. They need certain cofactors like zinc, copper, manganese, selenium, R-lipoic acid, and L-ascorbic acid, as well as several amino acids including (but not limited to) L-lysine, L-proline, L-glycine, and L-cysteine. Whenever the fibroblasts are unable to obtain the nutrients they need, the skin struggles because it cannot keep up with its collagen, elastin, and GAG needs that result from UV damage.

- **Macrophages** are unique in that they scavenge scar tissue and debris. They are also bacteria and fungi killers. In addition to that, they have the difficult job of manufacturing the vast majority of growth factors within our skin. This means that they are heavily involved in coordinating immune function within the skin. They are necessary for the repair and maintenance of the skin and its capillaries, as well as helping to regulate collagen and elastin production. I like to think of the macrophages as the "managers" of the dermis because they likely direct many of its activities, including lymphatic drainage, cellular repair, production of new capillaries, and the routing of nutritional components needed for the epidermis.

Every day there is a finite delivery of nutrients based on the amount of blood flow, how dilated the blood vessels are, how much cortisol is in the system, and other factors. All of these factors impact how many nutrients the skin receives. As we age, less and less oxygenated blood passes through the dermis, and more and more of the capillaries that are responsible for transmitting nutrients become increasingly damaged. This reduces the delivery of nutrients and provides another obstacle to maintaining enough nutrients to prevent the skin from thinning.

SUBCUTIS. The subcutis resides below the epidermis and is a source of stem cells, vitamins, minerals, and cellular components. Due to its depth, UV damage to this nutrient storage facility is less common. Fat cells also store toxins from our diet that can be dumped into the hair follicle to be excreted. The subcutis often contributes to cellulite because it swells from bad dietary habits in areas where the skin has "septae" that anchor it down. The result is the dreaded dimpling effect.

Great Adaptations

The skin adapts to an amazing variety of different environments. For example, over the many centuries of human evolution, we have seen that people who are born into more sun-exposed environments or geographies typically have darker skin. Africans, South Americans, and South Asians have developed the propensity to produce more melanin because their skin adapted to the climate that they were in. Although we usually talk about such adaptations in terms of generations, the skin does actually adapt during a lifetime. In fact, people with fair skin types who live in an environment in which they're exposing their skin to the sun on a daily basis will find that the skin will actually increase the number and workload of melanocytes in order to better prevent sun damage.

Skin also adapts to lack of oxygen. As years pass, our skin's metabolism slows down. Because of that, there is a declining need for oxygen. However if the skin is ever in a situation where it is low on oxygen, it will bring oxygen from the atmosphere to help maintain appropriate levels in the epidermis. Additionally, if the skin needs oxygen delivered to the epidermis, it will actually send a guardian antioxidant with it, because it knows that as soon as it puts oxygen into the epidermis, the sun will generate a free radical there. The companion antioxidant will squelch that free radical once it develops.

One of the skin's most important adaptations is its response to inflammation. When we go out into the sun, for example, the skin immediately starts manufacturing antioxidants and repairing damaged DNA that occurs as a response to exposure to UV light. This is a real-time repair effort, and each of us has a level of repair in waiting that is different—those of us with greater repair capacity can manage inflammation

Skin Malfunction, or Skin Smarts?

Sometimes we observe our skin's reactions and think we see disorder or dysfunction, when in fact we are actually seeing skin that is functioning properly. We can look to normal events in our daily lives for proof of this process. For example, when we stay out too long in the sun and we run out of our natural protectors like the stored antioxidants, amino acids, and cofactors that allow us to sustain and repair damage associated with UV light, we may develop a sunburn. Is that sunburn an example of the skin going haywire, or is it evidence of the skin's innate intelligence?

Redness from a sunburn does not occur because the skin doesn't know what it's doing or as a marker of defeat, but rather because the skin has put in a request to the body to say, "Listen we have sustained a great amount of damage here, and I need increased circulation so more nutrients and immune cells can be delivered to this area to improve the chances of a full recovery." The reason that a sunburn exists is because the skin is demanding that more assistance be provided to heal the segment overexposed to UV radiation.

Another example: When there's redness and swelling around acne, what we're seeing is an attempt to control excessive bacterial overgrowth. This is the proper action for the skin to take. With rosacea, the skin is experiencing a smoldering level of inflammation from an internal cause (most likely digestive). This puts increased demands on the skin, which result in increased circulation. The problem is not the redness in either of these two cases; the problem is the internal source of imbalance or the purposeful activities of healing skin.

better and will age more slowly and sunburn less often. This is different from melanin protection, which reduces the amount of inflammation inflicted. Others of us don't rely solely on our melanin, but rather we have very healthy antioxidant production levels that allow our skin to neutralize free radicals and prevent significant inflammation at the cellular level. This also allows us to extend our time in the sun without significant inflammation or damage.

Unfortunately, many of us have immunocompromised skin due to our diets, lifestyles, or the topical therapies we have elected to use. This results in the depletion of antioxidants and other protective and repairing nutrients. Any topical agent that interferes with the completed healthy epidermal barrier will promote inflammation and will further compromise, age, and endanger the skin. In a normal, healthy cycle, the epidermis would replace itself approximately every 30 days. What we have found is that, as we get older and as nutrient delivery diminishes, cellular DNA damage reduces efficiencies and manufacturing capacity diminishes. Instead of maintaining a 30-day cycle, our epidermis is forced to adapt, slowing its turnover rate to maintain a complete barrier.

To understand just what happens to our skin when we lessen its nutrient delivery, consider what happens when we starve ourselves: After only a few hours without food, our body recognizes that nutrients aren't coming, and it begins to slow down the metabolism of several cells within the body in an effort to preserve life. It figures that, in order to persevere through this loss of nutrients, it must slow down metabolism throughout the body so it can survive the shortage. In other words, it goes into survival mode. The same thing is true of the epidermis. When the epidermis isn't receiving the nutrients it needs—whether that's because of excess inflammation or the normal aging process—the epidermis adapts to maintain itself, knowing that without a full epidermal barrier the entire body could die from infection or fluid loss. Recognizing that there has been a loss of nutrient delivery, the epidermis slows its metabolism (and turnover rate) so that it can maintain a complete barrier without compromising the health and integrity of the skin. The skincare industry found that forced exfoliation speeds up turnover rate and understandably assumed that as an antiaging event. My view, however, is that the skin goes into an "emergency repair response," which means the skin isn't younger but rather more stressed and compromised from the exfoliation process.

Getting in the Way

Clearly the skin knows just how to take care of itself, and it does so in such subtle ways that the exact mechanisms remain a mystery. However, skincare professionals often misinterpret these adaptations and try,

Retin-A®

Retin-A® is a topical drug that is intended to mimic the retinoic acid manufactured by the skin. Retinoic acid is not stored by the skin, and so it is made in very scarce amounts whenever the fibroblasts are being asked to produce collagen. A certain component of skin cells that *is* stored (i.e., retinaldehyde) is often utilized to create retinoic acid. Retinaldehyde is pulled from fat cells or other storage locations and converted to retinoic acid in small amounts. The retinoic acid receptors on fibroblasts are then activated. When they are activated, the fibroblasts recruit amino acids and other mineral cofactors into the cell so that the process of manufacturing collagen, elastin, and GAG can begin.

unsuccessfully, to mimic them with one-size-fits-all approaches. But the skin has different and nuanced responses to different situations.

The greatest example of this is with the damaging practices of using daily acids, scrubs, or other exfoliating procedures. As I noted earlier, the ideal epidermal turnover rate is 30 days (meaning it takes 30 days for a keratinocyte to mature and become a corneocyte being naturally sloughed off). Procedures like exfoliation do in fact speed up that epidermal turnover by creating holes in the epidermal barrier that force the epidermis to go into survival mode, diverting nutrients from the (already deprived) dermis. Unfortunately, many skincare professionals just look at the end result—the hastened turnover rate—and see success. They mistakenly assume the skin is healthier, when in fact the reason for the epidermis speeding up its cycle has to do more with an emergency-repair response. The skin doesn't have the ability to repair the top sections of the epidermis without actually refurbishing the entire epidermis and processing all of the lower layers of the skin first. In order to create an intact stratum corneum or upper epidermis level, the skin actually has to send support from the bottom up in order to complete the renovation of the epidermis after it is damaged. In essence, the process speeds up to the detriment of the dermis, which could have used many of those nutrients to better maintain itself but instead had to divert collagen, antioxidants, and other components up into the epidermis. Remember that, while this is done daily anyway, forcing it to go faster when it has slowed for a reason means the nutrient shortages will only worsen in this environment. This does not even take into consideration the increased level of inflammation caused by the exfoliated skin. This puts even more stress on the immune system and depletes more components than if had we let the epidermis decide for itself the best rate at which to exfoliate.

Another example of the brain getting in the way of the skin is peptides. These are very popular ingredients in skincare products today. If you cut yourself and are going through a normal wound-healing process, there are different times when specific peptides are important and other times when they send the wrong message. So sometimes early on in a wound-healing phase, we will find certain growth factors critical to the progression of the management of that wound. At later times, that exact same growth factor is actually providing what we call a secondary feedback loop, meaning that it actually signals for the wound to stop healing. I bring this up because it makes it very challenging for us to try to guess when the skin would use a specific peptide or growth factor and when it wouldn't. In other words, while it may be totally appropriate to add a certain peptide at the beginning of wound management, using that same peptide a few days into the wound repair could be a confusing signal to give the skin. The obvious challenge occurs when we put peptides in skincare products because we apply them every day, even though it is likely that on certain days the product is sending the wrong message.

The same thing can be said of retinoic acid. Retinoic acid is a strong, effective signal for the manufacturing of collagen, yet large amounts of it floating around in the skin (as happens when people use products like Retin-A®) is not a normal physiologic event. It sends messages to different components of the remodeling aspect of the cell and actually interferes with the progression of normal epidermal maturation from a keratinocyte to a corneocyte. It even interferes with the process of tearing down damaged collagen at the dermal level and hinders healthy

Sun Sense

While various skin types tolerate sun differently, my opinion is that we are all designed to get sunlight on a daily basis. In fact, research shows that exposure to 15 to 20 minutes a day of sunlight significantly reduces your risk of developing several different cancers including colon, pancreatic, and breast cancer. This benefit is primarily attributed to the levels of vitamin D produced in the skin, but there may in fact be other beneficial aspects to sun exposure including the infrared waves. However, because of fears of skin cancer, premature aging, and other sun-related issues, many of us have gotten to the point where we believe sunlight needs to be avoided at all costs. I don't think that's true at all; my hope is that after finishing this book, you'll feel confident in exposing your skin to higher daily doses of sunlight without concern for any ramifications like skin cancer or premature aging. You can read more about my sun-care philosophies in Chapter 7.

melanin production. So while retinoic acid is very effective at its job, and it's very important that our skin makes it for us, Retin-A®, used daily on a long-term basis, can contribute to premature aging.

Ceramides are yet another example of skincare professionals misinterpreting the skin's normal functions. Ceramides are part of the lipid structure that creates the protective glue that keeps our epidermis functioning properly. They also function on a feedback loop. When we apply ceramides to the epidermis we are actually telling the cells at the base of the epidermis that they need to slow down. This is certainly not a message that we want to impart to the epidermis, because in most cases, people need their epidermal turnover rates to speed up—not slow down.

Let Your Skin Do Its Work

Examples like those above make it clear that, despite the fact that the skin is very adaptable, it can suffer from our interference. As good

~

The truth is, we are just scratching the surface of how the skin functions.

~

skin owners, we have to remember that the epidermis, because it is so dependent on the delivery of nutrients from the dermis, is susceptible to changes in its repair and maintenance functions, changes that depend on how healthy the blood flow is in the dermal layers. When a person smokes a cigarette, she experiences a massive decrease in the amount of nutrients delivered to the skin. This is probably one of the key reasons smokers typically age much faster than nonsmokers. In addition, stress (and the adrenalin and cortisol that come with it) impacts the delivery of nutrients to the skin. Caffeine may contribute negatively to the skin health by reducing its nutrient delivery through vasoconstriction. Once we focus on the keys to healthy skin, we can separate ingredients by their ability to enhance beneficial activities and eliminate the bad ones while taking immediate visible effects out of the equation. However, my experience is that the skin also shows visible improvement within weeks (if not sooner) of nourishing it properly.

The truth is, we are just scratching the surface of how the skin functions. However, from research and anecdotal evidence, we can clearly see that there are aspects to skin health and skin function that call for us to increase nutrient delivery to the skin, improve its protection mechanism, and analyze whether or not certain components are beneficial to the skin as a whole. If we trust in the intelligence of the skin and endeavor to work with—and not against—it, we will achieve the beautiful, youthful, and healthy skin we all desire.

To Sum It Up

Our skin is in a constant state of renewal and repair. But as we age, its normal functions become less efficient. To maintain its health as we grow older, we first need to understand how the skin works. The skin consists of three layers: the epidermis (the outer layer), the dermis (the middle layer), and the subcutis (the deepest layer). All the vitamins, antioxidants, and other nutrients that the epidermis needs come from the dermis. Some of the key components involved in this nutrient-delivery system are keratinocytes, which develop into the skin's protective barrier; lipids, those antiaging powerhouses that also protect us from dryness; melanin, which minimizes the damage from UV exposure; and stem cells, a good source of growth factors and repair regulation.

Many skincare professionals believe that the "dead cells" at the very surface of the skin are responsible for wrinkles, uneven skin tone, and dull, lifeless skin. On the contrary, this top layer is an essential part of a very carefully designed system and is in fact highly protective of and beneficial to the skin. Those so-called dead cells can actually prevent aging, infection, and dehydration, so they should not be forced off with harsh exfoliants and peels. In addition, this top layer of skin reflects 80 percent of damaging UV radiation, so when we exfoliate, a lot more UV damage can occur.

Our skin also suffers from the foods we eat and the stress we endure, depleting us of antioxidants and other protective and repairing nutrients. And the seemingly harmless creams we put on our faces and bodies to ease various skin conditions can actually cause inflammation and further age and damage the skin. But amazingly, the skin adapts to various environments and climates. One of its most important adaptations is the response to inflammation. Sometimes we observe our skin's reactions and think we see dysfunction, when what we are observing is skin that is working just right. Without a doubt, the skin knows how to take care of itself, but we must always be mindful that it is also susceptible to outside interference.

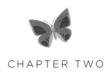

CHAPTER TWO

Skin Care Today:
Where We've Gone Astray

AS WE'VE LEARNED, THE skin is designed perfectly to function just as it should throughout our lives. Unfortunately, we tend to get in the way of the skin rather than aiding it in its natural processes. The myriad lotions, potions, and scrubs on the market just make it easier for us to do that. We entrust the skincare industry to tell us what's best for our skin but, for the most part, that approach has taken us down the wrong path. But before we tackle the question of how we've gone off track with our approach to skincare, it's important to take a look at where we've been.

Skin Care Through the Ages

Dating back to 4000 bc, humans used kohl, compounded from lead, copper, charred almonds, and soot, as makeup to emphasize and exaggerate the eyes. Substances such as milk, olive oil, nut oils, and herbs have been in use for millennia to nourish and improve the skin. Greek gymnasts applied olive oil before events to emphasize the sensual aspects of the musculature of the male form. By 1500 bc, the Chinese had developed formulas for painting the nails. Nourishing aspects of goats' milk were promoted, and botanicals had long been employed. By the time Cleopatra enchanted the Nile (69 bc–30 bc), it's not surprising that she took her milk baths with rose petals to improve her skin.

In the 1400s, fair skin became the desired aesthetic, and doctors and chemists concocted lead-based creams to sell to working-class women to hide the effects of the sun upon their complexions. Queen Elizabeth I (1533–1603) used a lead-based whitening cosmetic that, disastrously, led to mottling and disfiguration of her face. Nevertheless, lead remained a prominent cosmetic ingredient—despite generations of well-documented health problems—until 1869, when the American Medical Association published a case study on lead and palsy. Thirty-seven years later, in 1906, the US Food and Drug Administration passed the 1906 Pure Food and Drugs Act to regulate products that threatened public health.

Still, regulation of the cosmetics industry did not truly take place until 1938 and the passage of the Food, Drug and Cosmetics Act. The cosmetics business was still quite young but clearly showed signs that it would one day become a multibillion-dollar industry. It was during these early days that companies such as L'Oreal, Max Factor, Elizabeth Arden, Maybelline, and Revlon got their start.

A significant product appeared in the 1930s and 1940s that would change the way cosmetics companies thought about skincare: sunscreen. Developed by L'Oreal founder Max Schueller, this early sunscreen allowed users to take proactive control of their skin health. In 1944, a pharmacist from Miami, Benjamin Green, developed a special sunscreen for soldiers, who were being badly burned during World War II. The lotion Green developed was called Coppertone and it is still a top seller today.

During the past 30 to 40 years, the advent of alpha hydroxy acids, retinoic acid, lasers, and heat-based treatments has placed an emphasis on "rejuvenating" the skin. Unfortunately, in many cases, these methods do just the opposite. What all of these treatments have in common is that they a) focus on the skin from the outside in, and b) they actually accelerate skin aging. Nevertheless, technology and expediency are masters of the modern marketplace. Because the skincare industry has seized on these treatment approaches, it is heavily invested in irritating the skin.

As we know, the skin functions well when we don't interfere with its normal processes. But over the past 30 years, skincare philosophies have been focused on interfering with the skin's natural intelligence,

~

When you apply an acid to your face−
and this applies to almost
every acid, depending on the concentration−
you immediately create trauma.

⁓

and the results have been disappointing. The majority of popular skincare treatments today damage the skin and accelerate its aging, rather than delivering the antiaging benefits they promise. The reason? Many products and procedures that appear to reverse aging—by temporarily plumping the skin, lessening the appearance of wrinkles, and reducing color to the skin—in fact have the opposite effect. They increase free-radical damage, reduce the protective melanin in the skin, and starve the skin of critical nutrients and cellular components already in short supply.

The shift toward inflammation-inducing practices occurred around the time that retinoic acid was first introduced as an antiaging treatment. This also roughly coincided with the introduction of alpha hydroxy acids to aesthetic medicine.

Instant Gratification, Long-Term Detriment

The introduction of retinoic acid and alpha hydroxy acids to skincare products marks the first time consumers saw immediate gratification in their antiaging quest. It was a boon for aestheticians, who now had clients setting up monthly visits to get their acid fix as part of their facial. The results were impressive—plump, taut skin with a reduced appearance of wrinkles. Who wouldn't be hooked?

The problem, however, is that these results are only temporary, and in the long run they actually damage the skin and cause it to age faster than it would if we didn't use harsh products and techniques. The reason is that when we apply retinoic acid and alpha hydroxy acids to the skin, we are causing inflammation—and inflammation is bad for the skin. When you apply an acid to your face—and this applies to almost every acid, depending on the concentration—you immediately create trauma. This trauma results in swelling. Swelling makes wrinkles and fine lines look better, but only temporarily.

The other effect of these treatments is that they damage the epidermal barrier. The skin, being the intelligent defense mechanism that it is, sees this damage as an assault and seeks to fix the problem. In

Chemistry Lesson: What Is a Free Radical?

In chemistry, a free radical is an atom or group of atoms (such as a molecule or ion) that presents any number of unpaired electrons. In more understandable terms, it is an unstable "Tasmanian devil" that spins around looking for a stabilizer. In many cases, oxygen free radicals are taking electrons (to stabilize themselves) from DNA, cell walls, and many other cellular components. Webster's dictionary articulates why this is important to human biology. A free radical is:

An especially reactive atom or group of atoms that has one or more unpaired electrons, especially one that is produced in the body by natural biological processes or introduced from an outside source (as tobacco smoke, toxins, or pollutants) and that can damage cells, proteins, and DNA by altering their chemical structure.

Note the second half of the definition: Free radicals "can damage cells, proteins, and DNA by altering their chemical structure." The reason free radicals can have this damaging effect is that an unpaired electron is unstable and highly reactive—it's looking for a mate, and it bonds with the first electron it can in order to build stability. Free radicals, essentially, complete themselves by grabbing atoms from stable molecules, which can, in turn, become free radicals themselves. This sets off an atomic cascade of reactive behavior that is damaging to living cells. In fairness, free radicals exist because they make it much easier to make the reactions that keep us living. The real secret to all of this is that we are designed to deal what I call an "emergency repair response," the skin rushes to repair the damaged epidermis, which speeds up the epidermal turnover rate. Unfortunately, many skincare experts assume that increased epidermal turnover is a good thing—evidence that the skin is returning to its youthful functioning—yet, this forced exfoliation is actually the skin's equivalent of a four-alarm fire.

with this problem. The body is well aware of the threat posed by free radicals. This is why it makes a variety of antioxidants. The only time we get into trouble is when we exceed our repair capabilities, something much more likely to happen with the current exfoliation strategies being employed by most Americans.

To be sure, there's a vital exchange of energy associated with free radicals, and without them life as we know it wouldn't be possible. This is because of the process of oxidation that occurs during electron exchange. The body relies on oxidation to properly convert nutrients into energy. That's the upside of oxidation. The downside is that, inherently, oxidation is an act of decomposition or aging. Oxidation, after all, leads to rust. We've all seen cars so deeply affected by rust that it's a wonder the doors stay attached at all.

Now imagine all this activity on the surface of your face. Chemical exfoliation doesn't merely peel away the dead skin cells at the outer layer of the epidermis. Exfoliation actually upsets the atomic makeup of our skin, loosing a fury of free radicals that run around seeking stability and causing chain reactions at the atomic level. This eventually take a toll on the cellular makeup of the skin.

Let's sum up this chemistry lesson in three easy steps:
1) Exfoliation generates free radicals.
2) Free radicals lead to oxidation.
3) Oxidation causes our skin to age.

All of a sudden, it's easy to understand how unnecessary exfoliation goes against everything nature intends for our skin. All thanks to understanding the power and the danger of the free radical.

Increased Cellular Turnover and Melanin Production

As part of the skin's normal aging process, the epidermal turnover rate slows down to accommodate the declining availability of nutrients, cells, and other cofactors. Melanin manufacturing slows down as well. If you speed up the epidermal turnover rate by damaging the protective barrier, your melanin will not be part of the repair effort and therefore will not be available at the level it is meant to be. While this can be applauded as way to even skin tone by exfoliation, people are forgetting that the combination of an exposed barrier and reduced melanin leads to very unprotected skin, which will ultimately result in expedited aging and a worsening of facial discoloration.

Research shows that inflammation ultimately leads to a serious decline in the health of our skin. This can be illustrated by the broad array of different skin types, their melanin production, and their natural aging processes. Melanin provides natural sun protection to our skin— so much so that people with the darkest skin have enough melanin to provide a built-in sun protection factor (SPF) of 13.4. That means that sun exposure causes less damage—and less inflammation—in the skin of an African-American person than it does in a fair-skinned Caucasian. And it's no coincidence that, while people with light skin tend to begin developing wrinkles at the age of 30, it's not uncommon for very dark-skinned people to reach the age of 60 before they begin developing wrinkles. Simply put, less inflammation equals less aging.

This is not to say that dark skin does not experience inflammation and DNA damage. The difference is that dark skin has a greater ability to keep inflammation at a manageable level. Darker skin is still under attack by free radicals as soon as it is exposed to the sun, but it is better able to repair the damage—at least when it is kept to a modest level. Lighter skin types, on the other hand, accumulate so much damage (because their average, natural SPF levels are around 3) that the skin is unable to keep up—resulting in thinning skin and wrinkle formation.

Apply that knowledge to the use of acids: If we know that increased inflammation from sunlight alone can cause pale skin to age sooner than dark skin, just imagine how much adding acid-induced inflammation to the equation can accelerate aging!

The plumpness that results from the application of acids is not because collagen is being formed. The plumpness is a result of fluid accumulation. Whenever you create trauma in the body, the body increases fluid, which is needed to deliver the components necessary to fix the problem. True structural collagen changes take at least three weeks—well after the results from a peel have disappeared.

Nutrition and Skin Renewal

Over the past 30 years, many people have scheduled themselves for monthly acid burnings. It is important to understand that there is nothing gentle about alpha hydroxy acids when they are used in the strengths and pH levels currently being offered. They are designed to damage the skin. And yet, even though this is a rather barbaric process, we've been convinced that our skin needs it. What is the basis for that?

Among skincare professionals, there is a long-standing view that the best way to correct skin damage is to keep our skin cells turning over every 30 days instead of the 40 (or more) days we can expect as we age. The reality is that this is a prime example of our interference with the skin's innate intelligence. Our skin does not slow its turnover rate because it doesn't know what it's doing; it slows down because it is trying to maintain a healthy barrier.

When we think about the 30-day epidermal turnover cycle, there are a few questions that need to be answered. First, why does the 30-day cycle slow down? Second, why do 40-year-olds have a slower cycle than 20-year-olds? And finally, what is causing this slow-down?

My theory is that it's primarily about nutrition. Just like the rest of the body, the skin needs certain nutrients. If it isn't receiving them, the skin will go into survival mode. Think about what would happen to your body if you ate only 200 calories a day. Your metabolism would slow drastically, and all 50 trillion cells in your body would modify their behavior for fear of starvation. That's why you don't want to reduce your caloric intake too much if you are trying to lose weight. It will actually decrease your metabolism, and that would make it harder for you to achieve your weight-loss goals.

The skin is an organ in the body, just like all those other organs that slow down when they go into starvation mode. Every year of our lives, less and less blood flow is delivered to the dermis. As we know, healthy blood flow delivers nutrients (amino acids, proteins, enzymes, antioxidants, vitamins, minerals, and lipids) to the skin. All of those components have to be delivered or manufactured from delivered components on a daily basis. But, as our circulation decreases, our skin receives less and less nutrients. That leaves the skin with a choice to make: What can I modify in order to maintain life and protect myself? How do I best maintain the survival of this body? Believe it or not, the choice to slow the epidermis is a natural survival instinct.

When the epidermis thins, it is a life-threatening event. This is why we see such strong responses from the skin when we scrape, poke, or burn it. The dermis, on the other hand, can thin without disastrous results (although some people consider their wrinkles "disastrous"). Here's one way we know this: For the vast majority of people, the dermis thins at 1 percent per year starting in their 20s. Most scientists agree that this results from the overwhelming amount of repair demands placed on the skin. In our youth, we can handle the demands, but over time, we progressively see a decline in our immune function and nutritional support that leads to losses in the quality and thickness of our dermis. The epidermis, on the other hand, never really thins throughout our lives. In fact, if the epidermis were to thin at 1 percent per year like the dermis does beginning in our 20s, we'd likely die by age 50 as a result. The epidermis is unique in its ability to hold fluid inside the body and to minimize bacterial overgrowth and the absorption of environmental toxins. If that barrier were too thin, it would get to the point where we would be fully compromised and in a constant state of inflammation. Of course, that wouldn't matter much—we would undoubtedly die first from loss of fluids and infection.

Why is this important to understand? Because it fully explains what is happening in the skin. When the skin suffers a starvation event or starts to lose nutrients on an annual basis, it is forced to prioritize. It chooses

Reduce Your Epidermal Footprint

We think a lot these days about being green and reducing our carbon footprint. You can apply that same analogy to the skin. How can we minimize the amount of energy we are using to maintain the epidermis? The skin has already told us the way it does this—by slowing from a 30-day cycle to a 40-day cycle. Instead of trusting the skin, we say, "No, no, you didn't mean to do that; here's some acid to speed you up again." The skin doesn't thank us for this interference—instead, it thinks it's suffering an assault and rushes to fix the problem. As a result of the damage we have caused to the barrier, the skin must divert its limited resources and energy to fix an emergency of our own creation. Remember that the dermis is the one diverting these nutrients to the epidermis, so every time there are new demands from some procedure or application, it has an even harder time maintaining itself. Instead, we should tread lightly when we care for our skin, just as we aim to do on the earth, and trust in the intelligence of nature.

to forgo fully repairing the dermis the way it used to. And since it can't continue to provide the epidermis with all of the nutrients it needs to maintain a 30-day cycle, this slows the process down. As a result, the dermis is allowed to thin.

You can see how flawed it would be to assume that the skin does not know what it's doing when it slows down. From this new perspective it is easy to understand why forcing the skin to speed up this process through exfoliation can make the situation even worse. The skin is operating in an amazingly complicated fashion—much more complicated than we can understand—and it's doing a remarkable job. If we scrape our knee, it heals it. If there is some localized infection, it does its best to solve the problem. Epidermal tissue can sustain damage, and it doesn't matter nearly as much because it is almost always adequately repaired and replaced. That doesn't mean we should dismiss the damage as unimportant. Indeed, this damage comes at a cost.

Focus on the Dermis

The fatal flaw in our skincare approach is that we sacrifice the well-being of the dermis in order to keep the epidermis in a constant state of quick regeneration. We need to remember that exfoliation reduces the amount of pigment protection (melanin) we have and increases the amount of UV exposure, both of which increase free-radical damage and aging. This also causes dehydration and immunosuppression. In addition, it reduces our antioxidant protection, damages stem cells, increases the amount of DNA damage occurring in the skin (thereby increasing our risk of skin cancer), and it causes oil irregularities. It is a severe hit to the skin, but we continue exfoliating because we think it will improve our

The False Promise of Retinoic Acid

Retinoic acid (RA) is a perfect example of how harming the epidermis impacts the health of the dermis. When it came on the market, retinoic acid was touted as benefiting aging skin because it was proven to stimulate collagen activity in the dermis. Even today, it remains the most prescribed antiaging drug on the market. The funny thing is that, even though we have had 30 years to evaluate RA, the results are unimpressive. And, even though it *will* increase collagen production, the negative effects of retinoic acid overwhelm the positive with the end result being more rapid aging. I will be the first to admit that such a statement flies in the face of the current medical view, but I'm not sure everyone has been following the relevant research.

Retinoic acid, which occurs naturally in the skin in minute amounts, serves a significant purpose in the dermis—to stimulate fibroblasts, which make collagen and elastin. There are no fibroblasts in the epidermis, and their role there is limited and poorly understood. Research shows that when we apply retinoic acid to our epidermis, it doesn't just cause inflammation—it interferes with the epidermis' ability to complete a protective barrier by telling it not to evolve. It also interferes with the remodeling of the skin by telling the dermis to not remove damaged collagen. Do you see the irony in that? RA wrinkles. But you may be surprised to learn that our wrinkles are not a problem of the epidermis. Our wrinkles are created in the dermis.

It is dermal thinning and loss of elasticity that ultimately results in the formation of wrinkles. Even though it does little good to alter the protective epidermis, we have placed all of our attention on this visible layer of skin because it provides the most immediate gratification. Instead, we should spend our energy on the dermis. Until now, however, we haven't had the right technology to effectively do this.

Most skincare lines don't address the dermis. This is mainly because the majority of products only have a 2 to 5 percent penetration rate, which means most of the product stays in the epidermis. This damages

increases the amount of damage to collagen, and then prevents the skin from adequately removing the damaged collagen, which leads to structural collapse (thinning).

The skin doesn't store retinoic acid, because it is actually toxic to the body if it accumulates. Instead, it is created "on demand" so it can be immediately utilized. The body does this because there are only a few receptors that need to be activated to achieve collagen and elastin production. But scientists and physicians, having identified retinoic acid as one of the keys of aging, decided it would be beneficial to apply it to the skin. Unfortunately, they didn't take into account the fact that when you use retinoic acid on the top of your skin it damages your epidermal barrier. This, in turn, damages your collagen—which ages you further.

You can see how well-meaning people would recommend RA to reverse aging. After all, when you put RA on your face, it swells the skin and causes wrinkles to look better. But you can also see how long-term use of RA is anything but an antiaging event. In fact, I see people's skin looking older and less healthy as a result of using retinoic acid on a daily basis. If you put aside the fact that retinoic acid stimulates collagen and elastin, this makes sense. After all, each application damages collagen and elastin, generates free radicals, promotes inflammation, and strips the skin of nutrients. And yet, no one has questioned this popular "antiaging" strategy—until now.

the epidermis, resulting in a plumping of fine lines. Let's make sure that is clear: Most skincare lines have very little antiaging benefits (or other benefits), because their active ingredients cannot make it down to the lower epidermis/upper dermis. So these skincare lines, instead of improving delivery, focus on the epidermis, since inflammatory agents make us look younger when applied to the epidermis. Again, this is not true antiaging therapy; this is epidermal plumping. Antiaging products make improvements to the dermis, where the thinning actually occurs. Unfortunately, epidermal improvements disappear when the product is discontinued. Remember that collagen that is deposited in the epidermis does not correct existing losses to the dermis. This is also true regarding most chemical peels. Since they primarily burn the epidermis, there is no improvement in the layer of the skin that is actually causing the wrinkle (the dermis). In fact, burning the entire epidermis causes a massive diversion of nutrients and immune activity from the thinned dermis to temporarily help the epidermis.

Vitamin C and Collagen

Another acid used in a wide variety of skincare products is L-ascorbic acid, more commonly known as vitamin C. It made quite a splash, not only because it lends a "natural" feel to a product label, but also because it has been shown to stimulate collagen production. It's important to note that L-ascorbic acid does not function in the same way as retinoic acid, which prompts the fibroblasts to produce more collagen. Instead, L-ascorbic acid helps prepare the skin's amino acids for manufacturing collagen. When we don't have enough vitamin C in our diets, we don't have the component in our cells needed to put peptide chains together. This means we aren't creating adequate collagen (among other things), and therefore our skin begins to develop wounds.

But, like retinoic acid, L-ascorbic acid plays a very small role in the epidermis. The penetration rate to the dermis (where it's utilized for collagen production) is only around 2 percent. That means that when you put on a vitamin C cream, 98 percent of the active ingredient stays in your epidermis. This causes inflammation, irritation, light sensitivity, and exfoliation while also increasing free radicals. These are all the

More Is ... More

Because these ingredients have a poor penetration rate to the dermis, skincare manufacturers have sought to compensate by upping the levels of retinoic acid, alpha hydroxy acids, and Vitamin C. If 5 percent is good, then 10 percent is better, right? And if 10 percent is better, then 20 percent must be amazing! While it is true that more swelling can temporarily make lines look even better, the additional inflammation negates any potential benefit. As the industry keeps coming up with new acids to put on our skin, they're ignoring the reality that inflammation-based skincare simply does not work. We are already losing the inflammation battle. We cannot keep up with inflammation as it stands today—that's why our skin thins as we age. Any time we incite inflammation, we thin the skin even more. It's simply common sense.

things we want to avoid if we're going to create a true antiaging effect in the skin. Clearly, our strategy needs to change.

But again, people see results from vitamin C. Their skin swells, which means their wrinkles appear to diminish. They are fooled into thinking that they are experiencing antiaging in the skin. Here's a good rule of thumb: Whenever you see changes in wrinkles in the first 24 to 48 hours, you are not seeing changes in collagen production; you are seeing changes in the amount of fluid in that area. The epidermis is thinner than the edge of a credit card, so when you put something on it that causes inflammation, your wrinkle will *look* better—despite the damage caused to the rest of the skin. There are three keys to vitamin C: Do not apply so much to your skin that it causes it to become inflamed or over-exfoliated; make sure it has a delivery system that improves the 2 percent penetration rate; and make sure the product provides the components, in particular amino acids, that ensure the vitamin C is fully utilized at the cellular level.

One form of vitamin C, ascorbyl palmitate, was touted heavily a few years ago. It penetrated better, but the problem with it was that it had much less activity in the form it was in, so the net effect was less than using vitamin C. The best way to use vitamin C is to keep it dry and add it to a liposomal serum that can deliver it fresh to the deeper skin. The only form of vitamin C that is recognized by the skin is "ascorbic acid," which is chirally correct, more active, and less irritating than regular vitamin C.

The Air We Breathe: Oxygen and the Skin

For the past 15 years, we have seen a push to add oxygen to the skin through the use of skincare products and devices. This is based on the very true (and very obvious) notion that our skin needs oxygen. However, it's yet another instance of good intentions with bad delivery.

The dermis needs oxygen for the health of the cells and maintenance of cellular activity. The epidermis needs it, too, but it's not as important to the outer layer as it is in the dermis. All your organs and muscles receive oxygen from the blood as it passes through arteries. In many cases, the skin is the last stop on the line before the blood circulates back to the lungs for more oxygen. That means the skin is often the last part of the body that gets fed. Oxygen is plentiful in the dermis, whereas the epidermis has much less capacity to handle oxygen, so it keeps a smaller amount on hand. This is done purposefully because the skin knows that every oxygen molecule will become a free radical when it is exposed to UV light. The dermis, therefore, provides antioxidant "bodyguards" with every oxygen delivery to the epidermis.

While most of the oxygen in the epidermis comes from the dermis, there's actually one other method of delivery. Research shows that some oxygen can be diffused from the atmosphere through the epidermis, depending on the need. So, more likely than not, when our body is faced with fairly significant oxygen deprivation (in a very high-altitude or extremely cold environment, for instance) the skin can pull some oxygen from the atmosphere in order to maintain full functionality. Oxygen gives our cells the ability to perform at a much higher level, when it is needed. However, it is also the No. 1 cause of aging. While I don't have the research to prove it, I think it's safe to say that, since the skin is taking in this oxygen on its own, it's likely sending antioxidants to protect it, too.

Now that we know how oxygen is used in the skin, let's take a look at how skincare companies are trying to capitalize on it. According to some skincare manufacturers, decreases in oxygen may be one of the reasons we age, and therefore we need to supplement our skin with oxygen. Benzoyl peroxide and hydrogen peroxide both started showing up in skincare products, with the promise of oxygenating the skin. Unfortunately, benzoyl peroxide causes the loss of protective antioxidants with every application. Why? Because it is a free radical. You are actually putting an oxygen free radical into your skin. No wonder antioxidants run to the rescue and get depleted in the process.

Hydrogen peroxide is somewhat different. It is what is known as a precursor free radical. That means that it is stable in its true form but, because it readily breaks into different free radicals as soon as it's exposed to UV light, it quickly becomes unstable. In fact, when the body sees a free radical, one of the common ways that it stabilizes it is by turning it into hydrogen peroxide. This means that we already have plenty of hydrogen peroxide in our cells.

I would argue that we would want as little hydrogen peroxide in our skin as possible because of the dangers that it poses. The skin knows exactly how much hydrogen peroxide is around, and it provides enough antioxidants to manage the damage it generates. This typically works well unless we get sunburned or otherwise harm our skin and create so much

The Slap Test

Look at yourself in the mirror and find a wrinkle. Now slap it—not too hard, because I don't want you to hurt yourself—and you will soon see that the wrinkles in the area you slapped will look a little bit better. The reason is that your body moves quickly to repair trauma. When you treat your skin aggressively with an exfoliation device or procedure, you're doing the same thing: harming your skin—even though your wrinkle may look better.

free-radical damage that the skin can't handle it. When we put hydrogen peroxide on our skin every day, we trigger a flood of free-radical activity that overwhelms our skin's ability to fully recover.

So why did skincare professionals think it was a good idea to put hydrogen peroxide on the skin? Once again, it causes inflammation and swelling within the skin, and, lo and behold, makes wrinkles look better. But again, it does not help the dermis, from where wrinkles stem. If anything, it negatively affects the dermis by giving it more inflammation to manage.

One other way skincare professionals have attempted to add oxygen to the skin is with oxygen-infusion devices. These oxygen devices add free-radical damage to your epidermis and are not advisable. But their appeal is understandable. What happens is that when you start blowing oxygen onto erythema or red skin, you cause what's called reactive vasoconstriction. In other words, the blood vessels constrict to limit blood flow. This makes perfect sense since oxygen is carried in the blood. When oxygen is infused or sprayed onto the skin, we deliberately create a reactive vasoconstriction—a protective mechanism if you will, which diminishes redness on the skin. We think that means it is anti-inflammatory, but in reality it is the opposite.

Although the dermis can benefit from more oxygen, the idea of forcing it through the epidermis is ridiculous. All you accomplish is an uptick in free-radical activity. The best way to increase oxygen in the dermis is to take deep breaths, exercise, and use ingredients that improve circulation in the skin.

Over-Washing: How Clean Is Too Clean?

Somewhere on the timeline since our caveman days, we have developed an irrational fear of dirt. The result? We clean our skin—way too aggressively. I may give the germaphobes a scare when I point this out, but we have a significant collection of dirt all over our skin all the time. Debris floats through the air and lands on our skin, where it takes up residence until it gets washed off. I know it sounds gross, but the reality is that our skin is designed to handle dirt without developing any complications or infections.

From a skin-health perspective, dirt is not a huge risk—just look at our kids' ability to go days without showers. Dirt will not create inflammation in the skin unless it causes an infection. Even with acne, it is rarely dirt or debris that triggers a pimple. It is the existing bacteria on the skin. On the other hand, over-cleansing can have an aging effect on your skin. This isn't just because many cleansers contain irritants like sodium lauryl sulfate, but because we strip our protective lipids each time we clean our skin. This increases the potential for UV damage and dehydrates the skin. Even oily skin types mistakenly think they should wash away their excess oil. That, unfortunately, triggers the production of more oil. So the bottom line is that, while we should all maintain clean skin, it's important to avoid the scrubs and aggressive cleansers that will ultimately age the skin.

At some point, we have to have a balance between how aggressively we clean the skin and how much we leave behind, so that we don't have free-radical damage. In other words, if I cleanse my skin gently and get 80 percent of the debris off, my skin will be fine. My lipid barrier is intact, my stratum corneum is healthy, my skin is hydrated, I am bouncing free radicals away, antioxidants are in full supply, my dermis is not being overtaxed, and life is good. But if I overdo it, I am going to remove some of the dead-skin-cell protection and more of my lipid base. I am actually going to speed the aging process.

Here's the Scrub: How Exfoliation Damages the Skin

Perhaps the most damaging development of the past several decades is the gospel of daily exfoliation. We've all heard the argument, which is convincing on its surface, that we need to slough off our "dead skin" in order to let the healthy, vibrant skin shine through. What's more, we've been told that exfoliation speeds up our epidermal turnover rate to what it was in our youth. To help us accomplish this, skincare companies came up with countless scrubs and brushes to rub away the top layer of skin, the stratum corneum.

By most professional accounts, the stratum corneum is useless, dead tissue. I couldn't disagree more. The skin has several components that provide protection, and one of the most critical is the "dead" skin that is the last barrier between the body and the outside world. It prevents bacterial overgrowth, prevents fluid loss, reflects light (resulting in less UV trauma to the skin), and it holds lipids in place so they can provide a water-resistant barrier. It's a phenomenal layer of tissue—and yet we've spent the past few decades attacking the stratum corneum as if that's the reason our skin is dull and wrinkled. Remember, the skin only gets rid of its "dead skin cells" when it is ready—by pushing them off after their replacements arrive at the bottom of the stack.

Of course, when you scrub away some of the layers of the stratum corneum—which is actually made up of about 15 layers—your skin does look temporarily better. Exfoliation irritates the skin, making it plump and flushed from inflammation, but it certainly does not make it younger. It's just another case of interfering with the skin's natural processes.

The skin designed the epidermis so it only kicks off the top layer of dead skin cells when the deeper layers have made its replacement. But when we step in and use scrubs, brushes, acids, and microdermabrasion to reduce our stratum corneum, we also reduce the lipids in our skin, trigger water loss, and increase free radicals for several hours—if not days—until the skin recovers from the loss. So, even though the skin may look a bit better after you exfoliate, you are forcing it into a 30-day (or even shorter) renewal cycle. This not only causes a need for increased nutrition, but a significant portion of the collagen being made in the dermis is being forced to the epidermis to fix the area you are scrubbing away.

To Sum It Up

Because of the developments over the past several decades, we are facing a situation in which the things that we are doing to our skin make us look younger temporarily. But these actions will end up causing long-lasting damage. If you stop all of these daily skin treatments, you will know within a few days just how healthy your skin really is. *Warning: The results are depressing.* You will find that your skin deflates and sags. In fact, it may very well have aged significantly because of all the things you have been doing to try and make it look younger. We need to change our approach and do things that work on the dermal level. We need to stop creating inflammation and compromising the health of our skin. If we can do that, we can actually make significant—and long-lasting— changes to our wrinkles and the other signs of skin aging.

Part 2

~

Be Good to Your Skin

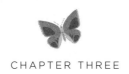

CHAPTER THREE

Common Cosmetic Procedures

IN THE PAST FEW DECADES, the fields of cosmetic medicine, dermatology, and aesthetics have exploded. Technological advances have made less invasive cosmetic procedures available and accessible to a greater number of people. However, we are just starting to understand the long-term effects of these popular procedures. It's time we re-evaluate their efficacy, safety, and overall effects on our skin health.

In this chapter, we'll explore three of the most common cosmetic procedures: lasers, chemical peels, and microdermabrasion/scrubbers. My hope is that after reading this, you'll have a better idea of how these procedures really work—and how they are failing to live up to their promises in many cases.

Lasers

Lasers have been used for several decades within the cosmetic industry, but the past 10 years have seen a significant rise in their popularity—in part because of their many available uses. While all of the new lasers on the market expand the possibilities for treatment, they also can be bewildering for physicians and patients alike. Here's a laser primer to help you sort through the different types, their uses, and their risks.

First, let's define what a laser is. A laser is a device that puts out a single wavelength of light. Each wavelength has a different chromophore, or target. A laser's use is often determined by how long of a wavelength it uses. The size of a wavelength is measured in nanometers; lasers used in cosmetic procedures use wavelengths from 300 nanometers up into the many thousands of nanometers. The vast majority of lasers range from 600 to 1,300 nanometers because those are the wavelengths to which the skin is susceptible that are capable of creating a cosmetic effect.

There have been significant advancements in lasers over the years. Some have been wonderful—for instance, ocular lasers have allowed doctors to correct cataracts and other vision problems. On the other hand, the fast and furious attempt to create newer, better aesthetic lasers has seen mixed results. Many of these lasers are highly touted using manipulated research from the manufacturers. This makes it difficult for physicians who use the lasers to sort through fact versus fiction. Some of my older, wiser physician friends who have been in the industry for a long time have a better approach: wait and see.

In the past decade, laser companies have made many amazing claims. But during that time, we've also seen companies rise and fall. A lot of physicians have also bought machines and soon regretted their purchase. Unfortunately, there is a lot of bad information surrounding lasers. As a result, physicians who are not knowingly or willingly trying to deceive the public end up making promises that don't hold true.

The average consumer gets a laser procedure done for one of several reasons:

- Vascular lasers treat visible capillaries, scars, and rosacea.
- Pigment lasers treat hyperpigmentation and remove tattoos.
- Antiaging lasers are used for collagen stimulation.

Vascular Lasers

Several different lasers can be used as vascular lasers, including those with wavelengths in the range of 532 nanometers and those with wavelengths of 1,064 nanometers. Both of these wavelengths are drawn to the depth and color of the blood vessels, so they direct their heat there. In addition, there is a device called an intense pulsed light (IPL) that employs high-intensity light using multiple wavelengths at the same time. All of these options have one goal in mind: to cause capillaries and/or veins to collapse, thereby reducing redness. Let's look at three of the most common uses for vascular lasers.

FACIAL CAPILLARIES. Visible facial capillaries, sometimes called broken capillaries, are one common reason that people seek out cosmetic laser procedures. Visible capillaries can occur due to physical trauma, overexposure to the sun, skin that has thinned from topical steroids or other reasons, DNA damage, and rosacea. Normally the blood vessels in our skin are fairly well hidden by the collagen matrix in the dermis. When our dermis thins, these blood vessels become more and more visible. Most fair-skin types develop them by the time they are 60, if not sooner.

When vascular lasers are used to collapse capillaries, the immediate effect in the skin is an inflammatory response. A blood vessel has been shut down and the body has gotten the message that an entire region of the skin is not receiving its nutrition or oxygenation. The body reads this as an emergency situation and begins the process of angiogenesis—the formation of new blood vessels—which takes about three days. The loss of local circulation may also result in atrophy (thinning) in the area as the cells die off from lack of oxygen.

With each passing year, blood flow to the skin is mildly to moderately reduced. This results in the typical signs of aging (e.g., wrinkles, visible capillaries). We are accelerating aging even more by using devices designed to shut down the food supply to a specific area of the skin. As we know, the skin is very well designed; it has capillaries feeding every part of the dermis. It also has excess capillaries in the upper levels of the dermis that feed the epidermis. The skin puts up with a lot of demand every day—we suffer a lot of damage from exposure to the sun and environmental toxins, It needs its full circulation capacity to meet those demands.

~

We are accelerating aging even more by using
devices designed to shut down
the food supply to a specific area of the skin.

~

Any time we cause an emergency repair in the skin, like we do when we use lasers to shut down blood vessels, we are robbing the dermis of resources it needs to sustain itself appropriately. Remember that the dermis is already thinning at 1 percent a year without these additional procedures; what do we think is going to happen when we cause an immediate regional loss of nutrients? My belief, based on what we know about anatomy and physiology, is that the dermis begins to atrophy for the three days before blood vessel replacements show up.

When an area of the body is cut off from the blood supply, it begins to atrophy. The cells without oxygen can try other means to stay alive for a period of time but, in general, they do not have the ability to adapt quickly enough and they tend to die. Affected areas (in this case, the dermis) most likely become thinner and actually lose some tissue. What's unclear is how much healthy new tissue is created once the blood vessel is restored three days later. We must also ask, how much is lost in the process? These are questions that need to be researched and evaluated more fully.

We also know from research that fibroblasts—the cells that are responsible for producing collagen—are very reliant on oxygen and blood flow. Any time we experience diminished circulation in an area, chances are good that we are losing fibroblast activity—and possibly even the fibroblast cell itself. So when we cut off blood supply by using lasers to collapse capillaries, what will the overall effect be on collagen production?

The simple truth is vascular lasers are not doing anything that promotes health or well-being in the skin unless you are collapsing vascular abnormalities like hemangiomas. Vascular lasers are often creating an aesthetic improvement in the skin, and the loss of a few capillaries spread around the face is probably an acceptable tradeoff. I get nervous when someone is collapsing 20+ capillaries at a time for all the reasons stated above.

SCAR TISSUE AND STRETCH MARKS. Another use for vascular lasers is to lighten scars and stretch marks. I have personally experienced scars with prolonged redness for several months. I have also had many patients with persistent stretch marks, and I certainly understand why people would want to eliminate them. However, laser

Are Those Capillaries Really *Broken*?

You've probably heard the term "broken capillaries" used to refer to capillaries that are visible. In reality, those capillaries are not broken— if they were, the blood in them would leak out into the skin and form a bruise. So "broken capillaries" is really a misnomer. Most of the time, capillaries are visible not because they're damaged, but because there has been a loss in the collagen that was hiding them from view.

treatments for these conditions take the same approach as those used for visible capillaries: They shut down blood vessels to make the redness disappear.

Again, we have to consider normal anatomy and physiology when deciding whether we should reduce the erythema (redness) associated with stretch marks and scars. Erythema is a natural part of wound healing. It is your body's way of providing blood to the area, this blood delivering the immune cells and nutrients needed to repair any scarring.

Our skin is constantly repairing wounds from sun exposure, acne, trauma, and aggressive procedures. It is normal for those wounds to take about a year to heal. Acne scars are a good example. If you have red acne scars on your cheeks that just won't go away, you may be tempted to consider laser treatments to destroy the blood vessels causing the redness. Lasers are quite successful at reducing erythema, and once it's gone, it won't come back. But when you use a laser to treat a scar, you are shutting down the skin's natural repair process before it has finished its job. This will obviously decrease the efficacy of the final phases of wound remodeling. As a result, the aesthetics of the scar will vary.

Just as we saw with the treatment of visible capillaries, we run the risk of causing atrophy when we use lasers to interfere with erythema. When we do not get an adequate replacement of healthy tissue in an area, over time the damaged collagen can continue to collapse. This will create cavities within the skin. These cavities take the form of stretch marks, which often become a cavity on the skin layer. We see the same thing with acne scarring as some acne lesions become pitted.

There are also many scars that do not benefit from laser treatment—it depends on the stage of wound healing and the type of scar being treated. It's important to be aware that there can be negative consequences when you collapse capillaries during the healing process. Although there is no published research, to date, that measures dermal thickness before and after a vascular laser procedure, I have seen a case where a patient lost a portion of the tip of his nose after shutting off a blood vessel in the region.

ROSACEA. The third and final use for vascular lasers is rosacea. Rosacea has been diagnosed in about 16 million Americans, but it likely affects twice that number. It is a chronic condition that results in redness, usually on the cheeks, nose, and forehead, and that comes and goes in flare-ups. Over time, the redness becomes ruddier and more persistent, and often results in visible capillaries and scarring.

I'll go into more detail about rosacea in my coverage of skin conditions, but I should mention that I don't think rosacea is caused by a skin problem. Yes, it involves specific skin signs, but I believe it stems from internal issues. However, in the world of conventional dermatology, attention is paid to the face since this is where the cosmetically unacceptable events occur.

At the skin level, rosacea is mainly a condition that involves chronic, smoldering inflammation. Whenever you have this kind of inflammation in the skin, you have huge nutritional demands. The body's response to these increased nutritional demands is to vasodilate, or open the blood vessels in that area so more nutrients and immune cells can be delivered. That is the first thing that causes the redness associated with rosacea.

A secondary event that worsens rosacea symptoms is dermal thinning, which results from chronic inflammation. Any time you have chronic inflammation in the body, the tissue in the affected area begins to atrophy (remember: The dermis can't maintain itself when it is constantly trying to put out fires and repair damage).

A person with rosacea seeking laser treatment might have up to 40 visible capillaries on the face. Standard treatment protocol has been to use a laser or IPL to shut these blood vessels down. For the most part, the lasers are very precisely targeted and attack only the blood vessels they are directed at. However IPL, which is also used for rosacea, doesn't just put out one wavelength. Depending on the type of head that's used on the laser, it may put off 10 to 100 different wavelengths at the same time. This means the heat generated by the laser can diffuse, because each of these wavelengths targets a slightly different aspect of the skin. You are also targeting a variety of depths of vascular capillaries—including some you can't see. This can potentially affect blood vessels that weren't visible and had no reason to be shut down.

Of course, with either approach, a significant number of blood vessels are being destroyed. This stops blood flow and nutrient delivery in those areas for at least three days. Rosacea sufferers especially need healthy circulation. Their inflamed skin desperately needs immune repair, nutrients, mineral cofactors, lipids, enzymes, and proteins—and in much higher doses than normal to keep up with the inflammation-repair process. Skin with rosacea has needs that are so significant that the body is actually dilating the blood vessels in order to bring more blood to the area. I believe that other modalities should be tried before considering vascular lasers when treating patients with rosacea. While lasers may make the skin look better by closing visible blood vessels, they impede repair of the inflamed skin.

Pigment Lasers

Pigment lasers use wavelengths that target darker colors in the skin. They can be used either to treat hyperpigmentation or to remove tattoos, and several options are available, depending on the problem being addressed. These lasers usually use wavelengths in the 500 to 1,200 nanometer range. They work by heating up the brown color you're looking to remove from the skin and essentially separating it from the basal membrane of the epidermis so that it will slough off. Alternatively, pigment lasers can heat the colored areas of tattoos enough to stimulate the immune system to carry the foreign material away. Since the laser is targeted to specific colors, it usually only has moderate effects on the surrounding skin. However, it is still damaging enough that people undergoing treatments for tattoo removal often suffer permanent scarring. Treatment for hyperpigmentation, on the other hand, requires fewer treatments, is more superficial, and is therefore safer.

People with darker skin may be at more risk because the laser will have a tough time differentiating between the targeted color and the rest of the skin. This can cause some heat damage to the surrounding areas. Patients with light skin will have a hard time removing light-ink tattoos (white, yellow) for the same reason.

Potential risks of pigment lasers include scarring, increased pigmentation, and hypopigmentation (permanent color loss).

Antiaging Lasers

When scientists were designing lasers to combat the signs of aging, they tried to determine which ones could stimulate collagen. What they found was that many different wavelengths stimulated collagen production. This may sound like good news, but to understand whether this is an appropriate and healthy use of lasers, we need to look at exactly how they trigger the production of collagen.

There is no question that the majority of "antiaging" lasers on the market today produce visible aesthetic responses in many people. However, as is the case with so many "antiaging" cosmetic procedures, the treatments do not seem to create an actual rejuvenating event in the skin. I realize that there's frequently supporting research that measures increases in collagen production or the reduction of wrinkles, but don't let that fool you. Anything that burns or wounds the skin will result in an increase in collagen manufacturing as part of the wound-healing response. In my opinion, collagen being made to repair a newly created wound (in this case, from a laser) will not be used to rejuvenate the original damage but rather be diverted to help the more immediate problem created by the laser. Doesn't it make sense that an increase in collagen production directly after a trauma means that the skin is making components to repair the newfound trauma?

The dermis has two responses to the heat and/or light of a laser: initial swelling and long-term retraction. While both can have cosmetic benefits, both are rarely a permanent reaction to the procedure. When we become inflamed from a laser treatment, the lines look better for a few days as the body attempts to heal the damage and the tissue begins to retract, which can also create a cosmetic benefit. Both reactions may

~

The average wound only recovers to 80 percent
of skin's normal capacity.

~

make fine lines look better and help soften scarring. In that regard, they are rejuvenating. Over time, however, the wounds heal and the skin is no longer swollen or retracted. This happens within a year. If the laser or heat device was aggressive, it might take a year before results disappear. Less traumatic procedures heal (results go away) within six months or less. I know that the laser companies would like us to believe that our skin looks 10 to 20 years younger after a laser treatment, but the evidence suggests otherwise. If a procedure really reversed aging by 20 years, then it would be unlikely that your skin would age the equivalent of 20 years in just six months. That just doesn't make sense. The other thing that does not make sense is that if these laser procedures really made our skin younger and healthier, then we would and should repeat these procedures over and over until we looked 20 again. Instead, laser and heat-based rejuvenation therapies are not cumulative. You often worsen results by trying to add more laser heat to an already treated area.

Bear in mind that repaired skin never quite regains its original health. The average wound only recovers to 80 percent of skin's normal capacity. That makes the decision of whether or not to wound the skin to reduce the signs of aging a tough one. On one hand, we like the effects that wounding creates: the lessening of wrinkles and increased firmness. On the other hand, will you be one of the many patients who does not fully recover from the wound?

Overall Laser Assessment

My overall concern with lasers is that they are often used too aggressively. Laser proponents have found that the more severe the burn, the longer the visible results last. Of course, you need to remember that the more aggressive you get, the more likely the possibility of severe, permanent complications. And most importantly, the lasers may not be doing as much good to the skin as you think. Burning the skin, and

Ablative Lasers

The term "ablative" comes from the word "ablate," which means "to vaporize or cause to evaporate." Ablative lasers belong in their own category, because they work differently than the other types of lasers we've discussed here. Ablative lasers burn off the top surface of the skin to cause it to resurface. In the process, this reduces fine lines and wrinkles. Erbium lasers and CO_2 resurfacing lasers are the two most common types of ablative lasers.

Erbium lasers cause much less heat damage, but do burn away the surface of the skin. Proponents claim much faster healing times and much less inflammation than with the CO_2 laser. On the flip side, the results are less impressive. Erbium lasers are more effective at treating fine lines than deep wrinkles.

CO_2 lasers are much more aggressive. In essence, they function as ablative lasers on the top layers of the skin, but they also address prominent wrinkles and acne scarring with heat that reaches into the deeper layers of the dermis. The result is a wound that can take as much as a year to heal. Aesthetically, there are some clear potential benefits to annihilating that amount of skin, but the risk from the procedure is pretty high. Many times during CO_2 resurfacing, the skin is damaged enough to actually prevent new pigment from being created, a condition called hypopigmentation. In fairness, the deep wounding effect can show dramatic improvements that are slower to disappear than most other laser treatments.

Despite its risks, I think there's a place for the CO_2 laser in the case of severely damaged skin (for instance, serious acne scars or facial laxity) as a potential alternative to a facelift. The key aspect of your decision to choosing a laser treatment is whether your skin can respond well to the trauma. For example, if you have serious laxity in your skin, that is an indication of a problem with your immune system and collagen/elastin production. Massive trauma to the skin could overwhelm the repair process and lead to severe complications. Similarly, if smoking is what aged your skin and you are still smoking, I would not advise performing deep peels or laser treatments.

thereby distracting it from its real purpose of maintaining itself
a healthy event. On the other hand, the people have voted and
clearly a popular option even though their results fade.

Heat Devices

Heat devices use radio frequency, ultrasound, and LED, along with other
methods, to generate change in the skin. Radio frequency, in particular, creates inflammation and subsequent tightening in the skin as it attempts to
repair itself. Even the medical industry has found some of these devices to
be too aggressive, and their use is on the decline. There are milder heat-gen-
erating devices that produce less impressive temporary results; but because
any effects from these heal more rapidly, the results do not last as long.

Ultrasound and LED are devices that add heat but not to the level of
trauma. Ultrasound can benefit the skin by improving nutrient delivery
by increasing circulation. LED does that, as well, but there is an instance
where diode lights actually trigger wound healing and collagen production. The key to LED therapy is exposure. If you are using a well-designed
LED light that uses a plate of lights that sit in front of your face then you
need one to two visits a week for 20 to 30 minutes at a time. If you are
using a well-designed handheld device, you should use it five days a week
directly on the skin for around five minutes per spot to see good results.
I have seen aging improve dramatically with this strategy. It is one of the
most cost-effective (and safe) antiaging approaches on the market.

Chemical Peels

Chemical peels, also called *chemexfoliation*, are extremely common in
the skincare industry. Chemical peels involve application of a chemical
solution that burns the top layers of the skin. They are used to treat fine
lines, mild scarring, acne, and hyperpigmentation.

Chemical peels have become the mainstay of America's current philosophy on how to rejuvenate the skin—as flawed as that philosophy may
be. They were born from the idea that the skin needs help with cellular
renewal and regeneration and, in particular, the renewal of epidermal layers. When we apply acid to the epidermis and cause its top layers to melt
off, we are forcing the process of epidermal turnover. As we discussed in

the previous chapter, this interference with the skin's natural functioning causes inflammation (with a side benefit of immediate aesthetic results). This also causes the dermis to divert its valuable resources to restoring the compromised epidermis. If the peel is damaging enough, the skin can require up to four times the nutrients normally needed to repair the barrier during the week after treatment. This is exactly the wrong approach. Robbing from the dermis to pay the epidermis only leads to accelerated aging in the long run since the dermis is where the signs of aging occur. Still, chemical peels have led to a massive increase in the number of skincare procedures done in America and throughout the world, so it's important that we understand what they are and how they work.

～

Robbing from the dermis to pay the epidermis will only lead to accelerated aging in the long run since the dermis is where the signs of aging occur.

～

Chemical peels use some kind of an acid, ranging from very low-strength glycolic peels, to phenol peels (the most aggressive on the market). As you might imagine, the overall effects of the peels can be very different, but the vast majority are designed to do one thing: burn off the top layers of skin and cause inflammation. Peels fall into three broad categories: mild/superficial, medium, and deep (see chart on facing page for a breakdown of the risks and uses of each).

Mild or superficial peels affect only the stratum corneum or a few of the lower layers of the epidermis, while the more aggressive peels penetrate deeper into the skin. Depending on the level of damage inflicted, you may see improvement in the visible signs of aging for anywhere from one or two weeks, to a year or more. There is a range of trauma levels, and being informed is the only way to know what to expect. Find out the type of acid being used, what the concentration is, and what the pH level is. Results also depend on the state of your own skin: If you undergo a peel when your skin has recently been exfoliated, the acid will behave even more aggressively and create even more inflammation. The bottom

TYPES OF CHEMICAL PEELS

Category	Chemicals Used	Uses	Risks/Side Effects	How Long Effects Last
Superficial Peels/Mild Peels	Glycolic acid Salicylic acid Lactic acid L-ascorbic acid Retinoic acid Jessner's Solution Retinol Facial Infusion™	Slight reduction in the signs of aging and sun damage; improved appearance of pigment changes, acne scars, and fine lines	Mild/moderate burning, redness, and peeling	About 1-2 weeks
Medium-Depth Peels	Trichloroacetic acid (TCA)	Creates second-degree burns to reduce the appearance of mild to moderate wrinkles, sun damage, and pigment issues	Pain during the procedure, swelling, crusting/flaking	3-6 months
Deep Peels	Phenol	Creates a deep second-degree burn to reduce the appearance of severe sun damage, wrinkles, pigment issues, lesions, and growths	Severe pain requiring anesthetics, extreme redness lasting 3 weeks to 2 months, swelling, infection, crusting, hypopigmentation. Rarely: heart, liver, or kidney failure	6-24 months

hat peels, like lasers, often create wounds to stimulate collagen and elastin, which means there is no net gain from the procedure, only temporary improvements created by swelling.

Facial Infusion™

This is my favorite option for an antiaging procedure. It really is not a chemical peel in the traditional sense because it does not contain the types or percentages of acids normally used, so it does not wound the skin. Instead, Facial Infusion™ uses 2 percent retinaldehyde, an ingredient proven in research to be similar to retinoic acid in collagen stimulation but much less inflammatory. That, along with 23 other ingredients, including 7 other research-proven collagen stimulators, is combined in a liposome delivery. It is often used alone and results in three days of peeling on average from the stimulation. Many physicians have used it with other treatments like laser or even harsh chemical peels to improve collagen activation. Facial Infusion™ is gentle enough for all skin conditions. I know the fact that most people peel from this treatment goes against my philosophy somewhat, but I believe that a few days of compromised skin is worth it for the many benefits Facial Infusion™ provides to the skin.

Microdermabrasion

The theory behind chemical peels is that the outermost layer of our epidermis needs to be removed in order to keep skin young. This is also the hypothesis behind another popular skin treatment: microdermabrasion. Microdermabrasion is a relatively painless procedure in which the stratum corneum is partially or completely scrubbed off using jets of aluminum oxide crystals or other components. People turn to microdermabrasion to treat sun damage, scarring, and hyperpigmentation. It has become so popular that home microdermabrasion kits are available to scrub away the skin and remove the stratum corneum.

Just like chemical peels, abrasive procedures can cause significant inflammation. Unlike chemical peels, most of the inflammation is not from the initial procedure but rather from the increased UV exposure that results. Microdermabrasion, scrubbers, and daily exfoliation generate free radicals that can damage the skin and reduce antioxidant activity.

~

We should be holding that barrier up
in reverence and protecting it.

∾

They also cause a loss in the ability of the skin to repair itself, so the effects can be doubly devastating. With the dramatic rise in skin cancer rates across the board, it is clear that we need to be much more careful about how many free radicals we expose our skin to.

Remember that darker skin has a natural SPF of 13.4, which can help postpone wrinkles for up to 30 years compared to those with lighter skin. Plus, the skin cancer rates in African-Americans are extremely low. These benefits are due to a daily reduction in free-radical damage from the sun. If you could prevent the daily bombardment of free radicals to the level attained with a natural SPF 13.4, then your skin would thin at a much slower pace and you wouldn't develop wrinkles until age 60. So why on earth would we want to use a scrubbing procedure to compromise the skin's barrier and increase free-radical activity? If a healthy barrier is SPF 3 in Caucasian skin, then we should start looking at an exfoliated barrier at "SPF -10." Microdermabrasion has a damaging effect on sun-exposed skin because it compromises the barrier more than we do when we use baby oil as a tan-enhancer. Instead we should be holding that barrier up in reverence and protecting it. After all, it supports every aspect of skin health and is one of the key ways that we keep the inflammation to a minimum. It is also one of the key ways that we prevent skin cancer, fluid loss, and bacterial infection.

The second problem with microdermabrasion is that it dehydrates the skin by removing the lipids and the protein barrier in the epidermis. As we remove that barrier, we actually allow moisture to leave the skin. Since the skin below the stratum corneum is 70 percent water, that actually becomes a factor and that's probably why America as a whole is addicted to moisturizers—yet these products should really be unnecessary.

I understand why people think scrubs are a good idea. We look at the peeling, scaly skin on our legs and think we need to scrub it off. What

…don't realize is that the skin is not scaly because it failed to perform properly or doesn't know what it is doing; it's scaly because of chlorine in our water, hot showers, dehydration, and a variety of other things. The scales are actually the result of a damaged barrier, and yet our response is to damage the barrier further by scrubbing it. This is why we need to continually exfoliate and moisturize, even though neither of these measures solve the problem.

I suggest limiting or avoiding microdermabrasion and other scrubbing procedures, because they only work on your epidermis and they increase inflammation. Your epidermis is just going to become dust within 30 days of commencing its process, so there is absolutely no need to spend time or money on the epidermis, particularly if the time is spent damaging it and the rest of the skin.

Some People Still Want Their Fix

I have been teaching this philosophy for a few years, and the strategies have been used by many estheticians, physicians, and tens of thousands of patients. People have had wonderful results using my skincare line (Osmosis) and avoiding daily, forced exfoliation. I have great stories of estheticians who spent the last 25 years exfoliating and, with a leap of faith, quit exfoliating procedures cold turkey only to find better results than ever before. That being said, sometimes people just want an exfoliation of some kind, whether it is a procedure, an acid, or an enzyme mask. They often ask if monthly peels are such a bad thing. My response is this: Daily exfoliation procedures and exfoliating chemicals are a mistake. Weekly, heavy exfoliating treatments like peels will still age the skin. Monthly peels, if no more than a very mild acid, can be managed by the skin without significant losses to dermal nutrients or significant additional inflammation.

To Sum It Up

Most of these procedures that have transformed the field of aesthetics over the past 30 years have one thing in common: They cause inflammation. They may provide some instant gratification, but in the long run they will age the skin faster. Just look at the overall results of the last three decades of chemical peels, laser and heat treatments, exfoliants, and microdermabrasion. Have we stayed younger longer? No. In fact, I'd argue that the opposite is true. As I look at the skin of people who have had several traumatic chemical peels over the years or those who exfoliate or use retinoic acid daily, I find that their skin is thinner and more fragile. If they stop the peels and other exfoliating procedures for a few days to a week, they will find that, as the swelling goes down, their wrinkles look worse, not better. Instead of fewer visible capillaries, they may have more. Instead of more even pigmentation, the skin appears splotchy because the melanocytes have been damaged. Unfortunately, in the face of their skin's rapid decline, they will resume their old skin-care habits to get the plumping—a misleading side effect—back. But I'm here to tell you that you can repair your skin, in ways we'll outline in future chapters—ways that are healthy and nourishing for the skin, that work with the skin and not against it. The first step? Ending the exfoliation addiction.

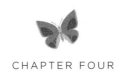

CHAPTER FOUR

What's in Your Makeup Bag? A Look at Popular Ingredients in Cosmetics

IN THE LAST CHAPTER, we talked about the procedures that are damaging to the skin. But even more pervasive are the harmful ingredients in skincare products. Virtually all of us use some sort of cosmetic products—whether they're cleansers, scrubs, moisturizers, or even just plain soap—that contain ingredients that are bad for our skin. Some of those ingredients cause inflammation. Other ingredients are suspected of contributing to serious health risks like breast cancer. That's why it's important that each of us understands what's in the products we use on our skin so that we can make the most informed and healthy choices possible. Below is a list of some of the ingredients I like and many that I think you should avoid. This is not a complete list by any means, so I focused on ingredients that I do not think are discussed enough.

Alpha Hydroxy Acids

Alpha hydroxy acids (AHAs) are a category of compounds, either natural or synthetic, that share a similar chemical makeup. Some of the most well known AHAs are glycolic acid, lactic acid, mandelic acid, and malic acid. Mild or superficial chemical peels, as discussed in the previous chapter, often use glycolic acid. In lower concentrations, glycolic acid and other AHAs show up in many everyday cosmetics.

AHAs in skincare serve a similar purpose to those in chemical peels—to hasten epidermal turnover ("exfoliate") and assist with issues like hyperpigmentation and fine lines. Of course, cosmetic products are much less traumatic than a chemical peel but they still result in inflammation. The skin reacts to different AHAs differently, so it's hard to make a blanket recommendation about whether to use them or not. For example, glycolic acid is not meant to be in or around the skin, so there is no point to using it unless the point is to force exfoliation by damaging the epidermis. Lactic acid is a different story. It is a natural moisturizing factor and is reported to have antioxidant properties. This means that lactic acid can actually benefit the skin.

~

In this age of skyrocketing skin cancer rates, it just makes no sense to do anything to the skin that reduces our skin's ability to protect itself from sun damage.

~

To be clear, there is some benefit from using lactic acid on the skin, but only in moderation (less than 5 percent in a formula). Mandelic acid can also help control bacteria if used in moderation. The key is not having a product that damages the barrier, and these two AHAs—used in low concentrations—can achieve that. Most products use AHAs at levels designed to exfoliate and traumatize because of the plumping that results, but I advise against using these products on a daily basis, and especially not at concentrations above three to five percent. At higher concentrations, AHAs burn the epidermis—and you are not going to rejuvenate your skin by doing that. In fact, your skin will age faster because the collagen needed to fix the burn in the epidermis could have been used to maintain or rebuild your supply of dermal collagen.

Neutralize It

You may encounter products with AHAs that have been "neutralized." This wording is intended to make you think you'll get the same benefits acids provide without the detrimental effects. Unfortunately, that's not the case. If an acid has been neutralized, it is no longer acidic. The good news is that it won't create inflammation, but the bad news is that it will not achieve its goals since acids need to create inflammation to plump the skin as intended.

Retinoic Acid

Retinoic acid is probably the most common skin prescription in the world. It entered the cosmetic scene 30 years ago when it was determined that one of the ways fibroblasts make collagen and elastin is through a molecule in the skin called retinoic acid.

The formation of retinoic acid is the last step in a chain of events that leads to collagen stimulation. It starts with beta-carotene, which is often converted to retinol. Retinol, in turn, can be converted back and forth into retinyl palmitate and retinyl acitate, the most commonly stored forms of Vitamin A. These forms can all be converted to retinaldehyde. Retinaldehyde is then converted to retinoic acid, which activates fibroblasts to create collagen. Retinoic acid is not stored in the skin; instead, tiny amounts are made within the dermis as needed for collagen production. The process is very careful and precise, because retinoic acid is actually toxic to the skin. You may be wondering how the skin can manufacture something toxic. Well, just as lactic acid is beneficial to the skin in small amounts but damaging in higher doses, trace amounts of retinoic acid can be very beneficial for the skin. When the skin has more than it can utilize, though, retinoic acid is damaging.

Applying retinoic acid to the skin topically becomes a challenge because, in high amounts, the epidermis misinterprets its presence. It sees the retinoic acid as an indication that there's something wrong in the physiology of the skin. The skin then sends a chemical message telling the keratinocyte (the main cell of the epidermis) that it should not mature to a corneocyte (a key reflector of UV damage). In summary, topical retinoic acid actually interferes with the normal maturation process (i.e., the normal turnover process) of the skin.

We also know that retinoic acid is exfoliating, so the daily use of it compromises the epidermis by removing the already beleaguered stratum corneum, as well as some of the lipid structure of the skin. This also triggers inflammation and increases free radicals substantially. Add to that the fact that retinoic acid stops the normal progression of the epidermis and we see even more severe increases in sun sensitivity. Here's a word of warning: Any product that creates "sun sensitivity" is, by clear definition, aging your skin because it means that you will suffer more sun damage as a result of using the product. And sun damage equals both aging and an increased risk of developing skin cancer.

The third problem with retinoic acid products is that they send a chemical message to the skin's metalloproteinases (MMPs) to stop tearing down collagen. Normally, when new collagen is formed, damaged collagen is broken down and eliminated. But retinoic acid interferes with this normal process, leading to a collapse of dermal structures. It's akin to building a brand new house on top of a bunch of decayed wood that has been run over by a bulldozer. The house will be unstable, and you won't be able to erect walls properly with all those extra wood pieces lying around. So when retinoic acid is applied to the skin in confusing amounts, it actually obstructs the skin's natural protection and repair process.

Often when experts discuss topical retinoic acid, they laud its ability to interrupt the normal dismantling of collagen as though it were an asset. They consider it an antiaging effect because it "prevents collagen

~

Here's a word of warning: Any product that
creates "sun sensitivity" is, by clear definition,
aging your skin because it means that
you will suffer more sun damage as a result of
using the product.

~

Oral Retinoic Acid

The oral form of retinoic acid, Accutane (isotretinoin), is frequently used for severe cystic acne. Over the years it has proven to be incredibly toxic to several organs in the body. It also inhibits wound repair. Accutane should be avoided if at all possible because of its detrimental effects on the liver, lungs, eyes, and skin, and its mood-altering effects like severe depression. That being said, Accutane is still frequently prescribed, so it's important that you do your own research before you allow your doctor to prescribe it to you or your child.

loss." But I would argue that it is, in fact, an *aging* event because it allows damaged collagen to hang around within the skin. Remember, the skin only tears down damaged collagen, not healthy collagen. This might explain why, when I look at the skin of people who use Retin-A® daily for a year or more, I notice that their skin looks thin and unhealthy. If Retin-A® really lived up to its promise, everyone using it would look younger every year. That is clearly not happening.

As a final blow to the skin, retinoic acid damages our protective melanocytes. The cytotoxicity of its presence reduces melanin, thereby increasing free-radical damage once again.

Hydroquinone

Hydroquinone is an ingredient used to treat hyperpigmentation. It does this by hindering the production of melanin. Hydroquinone is extremely common in the US market, but it is much less common outside of the United States because so many countries have banned its use. The reason? Serious risks, including cancer and organ toxicity. It can also cause a condition called exogenous ochronosis, a permanent bluish-black pigment stain in the dermis.

We also know that hydroquinone is toxic to melanocytes. Remember, melanocytes are the cells that produce melanin, the protective pigment in our skin. Every year of our lives, the number of melanocytes we have in our skin decreases naturally, which means we have less protection against sun damage. Adding hydroquinone to the equation just accelerates that process. In addition, hydroquinone is inflammatory to the skin, which hastens aging, as well.

Maybe—*maybe*—these risks would be worthwhile if hydroquinone actually corrected hyperpigmentation as it is professed to do. But it doesn't. Hyperpigmentation, especially on the face, can be a serious concern for many people, and they will do just about anything they can to make the discoloration go away. Unfortunately, hydroquinone is just a temporary fix with moderate results, which is why hydroquinone is often added to other ingredients to make it work better. Personally, I think it is the associated inflammation that stimulates melanin and makes the results less than perfect. Unfortunately, like most lighteners, it must be applied repeatedly, forever, to keep skin tone even. Many people experience a "rebound" of their pigment after discontinuing use because hydroquinone leaves a trail of inflammation that likely triggers more melanin to be produced. The bottom line is that hydroquinone ages the skin and is moderately toxic, so I am not a fan. The good news is that other, less risky strategies are available for treating hyperpigmentation. I'll address those in Chapter 9.

Steroids

Steroids are sometimes prescribed for skin conditions like dermatitis, psoriasis, and eczema. The intent is to mimic steroids' natural function in our body and control the inflammation process. Within the body, the steroid hormone cortisol is released in response to inflammation to slow down the repair process (at the right time) and prevent scarring. When psoriasis or eczema patients take steroids, either internally or topically,

~

Unfortunately, hydroquinone is just a temporary fix, which means it needs to be applied repeatedly, forever, to keep skin tone even.

~

the purpose is to interfere with the body's immune response. Steroids also reduce the amount of nutrients that are delivered to the site via the blood vessel walls. The combined effect of those two events leads to significant trauma, atrophy, and scarring with repeated use.

I advise avoiding steroids whenever possible. Instead, seek out medicinal strategies that work on the underlying cause of the condition rather than just blocking the immune system. Remember, even mild steroids age the skin so if you must, limit steroid use to as few applications as possible.

Antibiotics

Antibiotics are another commonly prescribed medication for skin conditions like rosacea and acne. They can be used either internally or topically. Antibiotics obviously have some definite benefits like temporarily reducing bacterial counts, but they also have drawbacks. Like steroids, antibiotics suppress the immune system, which may be a main reason that they can reduce redness in rosacea. They also kill off good bacteria and significantly affect the health of the digestive tract. This is a major problem for the entire body because the digestive tract is involved in the immune activity and many other aspects of day-to-day life.

But my main concern with antibiotics is their overuse. Overuse allows antibiotic-resistant bacteria to develop. Antibiotics can also enter our water supply. This is particularly true for topical antibiotics, which aren't absorbed well by the skin and are often washed off. Because of their effect on both the body and the environment, I think antibiotics are a last resort for treating skin conditions—especially since bacteria can be controlled with several less harmful compounds.

*Reducing blood supply is never a good way
to promote skin health, because it reduces nutrient
delivery to the skin.*

Vitamin K

Vitamin K has shown up in many creams over the past several years
with the promise of addressing under-eye circles and visible (so-called
"broken") capillaries. It works by promoting clotting in blood vessels,
thereby eliminating discoloration. As I explained in the previous chapter, I would rather avoid shutting down capillaries for cosmetic effect.
They have an important function—to deliver nutrients to the skin.
Preventing that task only accelerates aging and reduces our skin's ability
to handle everyday challenges. Therefore, I suggest avoiding vitamin K
in skincare products, especially under the eye where more nutrients are
needed, not less.

Caffeine

We all know the caffeine in your morning coffee can help you power
through the day when you haven't gotten enough sleep. But, what about
the under-eye bags that also accompany sleep deprivation? According to
several skincare manufacturers, all you need is more caffeine—applied
directly to your skin. Several products on the market today claim to
reduce puffy eyes, cellulite, and other signs of inflammation, and they
do have some effect. However, the way it addresses this inflammation is by constricting blood vessels. As I've explained, reducing blood
supply is never a good way to promote skin health because it reduces
nutrient delivery to the skin. I advise against using caffeine-containing
skincare products.

L-ascorbic Acid

L-ascorbic acid, also known as vitamin C, has numerous health benefits. In the body, it is essential for collagen synthesis, which is why

Devil's in the Details

The only form of vitamin C that is active in the skin is L-ascorbic acid. Products containing "Vitamin C" on the label contain two forms of the molecule: "l-ascorbic acid" and "d-ascorbic acid." Research shows that the "L" form is much better for the skin. When we use ingredients that have been purified to that level we call it "chirally" (pronounced *ki-raly*). Unfortunately, some companies go the cheap route and use a combination of plain Vitamin C, which is half as effective and twice as irritating. If you see the words "ascorbic acid" without an "L," move on to a different product.

Also, the absorbency of vitamin C can be increased with a technology called "liposomal delivery." What this means is the vitamin is encased in a lipid sac that allows it to penetrate more deeply into the skin. Ascorbyl palmitate, another alternative with better absorption, has been proven to be much less active in the skin even though it is a stable form of the vitamin and has better penetration.

skincare companies incorporate it into their products. But when it comes to skincare, vitamin C is a perfect example of how a good thing can go bad.

Most of the important work that vitamin C does occurs in the dermis. However, because of the way skincare products are designed, the vitamin is applied to the epidermis. Unfortunately, only about 2 percent of the nutrient penetrates down to the dermal/epidermal junction, which leaves a whopping 98 percent in the epidermis. While in the epidermis, vitamin C exfoliates the skin and also oxidizes—which means it creates free radicals within the skin. As we know, free radicals are a detriment to our health long-term. Vitamin C often is a plumping agent because of this limitation—which is why vitamin C-based products have enjoyed significant market success. The challenge is how to enjoy the benefits of vitamin C without inducing inflammation.

Because of vitamin C's poor penetration rate, manufacturers are practically tripping over each other trying to get the highest concentrations on the market. But the danger of higher concentrations is that they cause more oxidation and inflammation in the skin. If you are going to use a topical product with vitamin C, do not exceed a concentration of 10 percent and make sure it has an effective delivery system. I prefer delivering vitamin C in powder form and mixing it in a liposome serum right before application to avoid the inevitable oxidation that occurs in the bottle. Oxidized vitamin C is not nearly as beneficial as fresh, undamaged C—which is why keeping it in dry powder form is so helpful.

Peptides

The word *peptide* is a very general term that describes at least two amino acids that are joined together. A single amino acid is an amino acid, but two or more stuck together become a protein or a peptide. Peptides come in variety of lengths using varying amino acid chains. The bigger the chain of peptides, the less likely it is to penetrate the skin. Since larger peptide molecules struggle to get into the skin, I'm a fan of smaller molecules and even amino acids alone.

What is the purpose of including peptides in skincare? There are a number of claims, ranging from smoothing rough skin, to diminishing wrinkle depth and volume, to muscle relaxation. In most cases, the peptides in skincare are intended to mimic some sort of physiological process within the skin. For the most part, though, they do not have an antiaging effect because they get trapped in the epidermis. Although these peptides are usually modeled after those found in the dermis, skincare manufacturers have not done a very effective job of formulating their delivery.

One claim you'll often hear about peptides is that they effectively relax muscles. This makes them useful for preventing lines caused by repetitive muscle movements (like laugh lines). However, evidence suggests that that is an over-hyped claim and that peptides don't actually have a significant impact on muscle contraction. Instead, the tautness felt in areas with muscle-related wrinkles result from a buildup of peptides within the epidermal layers.

Peptides are also used for other purposes in skincare. There are reportedly peptides that reduce oil, and others that boast antioxidant protection, but these peptides primarily work by lodging themselves in the epidermis and creating a temporary plumping effect. The drawback to this is that the effects only last for as long as you keep using the product. Once you discontinue use, all the benefits go away. That is not true across the board, but it is true in a vast majority of cases. In fact, some skincare companies go so far as to combine peptides with other inflammatory agents to enhance the plumping effect. But again my preference is toward non-inflammatory plumping, which doesn't force epidermal turnover. Peptides, in general, are good, non-inflammatory plumpers. For this reason, peptides are an acceptable approach to the antiaging strategy as long as they are used with ingredients that really do correct damage.

Sodium Lauryl Sulfate

Sodium lauryl sulfate is a common ingredient in face washes and liquid soaps because it is a very effective cleanser. However, countless studies over the years have proven it to be a very strong irritant. In fact, when researchers are testing anti-inflammatories, they often use sodium lauryl sulfate to create the inflammation they'll then seek to combat. This hardly seems like a good choice for daily skin use.

The reason manufacturers continue to use sodium lauryl sulfate is because it lathers well and strips dirt from the skin—the two main things we're looking for when we're trying to get clean. But I'll argue again that a little bit of dirt is better for the skin than harsh chemicals. There's no reason to overcleanse the skin. When we do, we remove essential lipids from the epidermal surface and suffer far more inflammation than we ever would have had we simply left a little extra makeup on our face.

Parabens

Parabens, a class of chemical that includes methylparaben, propylparaben, and butylparaben, are the most widely used preservatives in cosmetic products. Most products use more than one paraben (you'll see them toward the end of the ingredients list) as a way to prevent spoilage from microorganisms.

Over the past 10 years, parabens have come under scrutiny in the scientific literature because of their estrogenic activity. Certain types of breast cancer are known to be dependent on excess estrogen in the body and, in 2004, researchers published a study in the *Journal of Applied Toxicology* noting that parabens were found in breast tumors. Since then, more studies have been conducted, with mixed results. Some industry representatives—as well as the US Food and Drug Administration— hold that the levels of parabens in cosmetics are too insignificant to pose a risk. Others are wary of such claims and would rather not take the risk.

I think there is too much evidence of their toxicity to feel comfortable having them in your skincare products. There are safer preservatives that should be used until we know the real consequences of using these ingredients. In addition, parabens tend to damage the expensive active ingredients in products, which means they can result in less active, less corrective skincare. Supporters of parabens always use the argument that it is better than having a bunch of bugs growing in the product. While I agree, they still miss the point: We have better options that are not toxic to the skin and body.

Ceramides

Ceramides, a family of lipids, are used in products designed to treat dehydration, eczema, and psoriasis. They're part of our natural moisture complex, the skin's lipid barrier. But when they are included in a moisturizer, they don't function as we may hope. When the skin senses that it has too many ceramides (which is what happens when we slather them on in a cream), it sends a message to the epidermis to slow down its turnover rate. Therefore, products containing ceramides can have a mild aging effect.

Glycols

"Glycol" describes a chemical compound containing two hydroxyl groups. The specific glycols that show up most commonly in cosmetics are propylene glycol, ethylene glycol, and polyethylene glycol (PEG). Each type has a different set of uses and a different safety profile—and some are safer than others. However, the overarching message about glycols is that, when used in a high percentage, they strip the lipids from the skin, increase free radicals, and dehydrate the skin. Propylene glycol is the worst offender of the group and should be avoided.

Oxygen

As I explained in Chapter 1, many skincare manufacturers are seeking to deliver oxygen to the skin through their products. You may see it in the form of benzoyl peroxide or hydrogen peroxide. The idea of using oxygen on the skin makes sense on the surface, since oxygen is hugely beneficial to the dermis and we have less of it in our skin as we age. But the truth is that the skin controls oxygen very well, and it is too dangerous a tool to use because of our inability to control its damaging effects. Topical oxygen can fool us. For example, it may appear that topical oxygen is anti-inflammatory since it causes the constriction of blood vessels. If you are experiencing redness on your face and spray it with an oxygen-based product, you may see the redness diminish. You may also see an improvement in fine lines since another reaction from the use of topical oxygen is plumping from inflammation.

The epidermis has a lower need for oxygen (by design) than does the dermis, because oxygen immediately becomes a free radical when exposed to ultraviolet light. This happens much more readily at the top layers of the skin. The skin combats oxygen free radicals with antioxidants because it needs the oxygen to survive. It is a very delicate balance. If you put oxygen onto the epidermis, however, you're actually putting free radicals into the epidermis. As we discussed in the previous chapter, when the skin moves oxygen from the dermis to the epidermis, it always sends that oxygen up with an antioxidant bodyguard. This doesn't occur when we add oxygen to the skin topically. Even if it did, those antioxidants would be better served fighting existing aging instead of battling the free radicals created when topical oxygen was applied.

Knowing that oxygen is fragile, I like to limit its use in skincare products and services. It is yet another example of a compound that can be beneficial in small amounts and harmful in excess. The bottom line is that the skin adjusts its oxygen level based on demand, and far be it from us to assume we know the exact oxygen demands of the skin. This is why these oxygenated topicals should be avoided.

To Sum It Up

Common cosmetics seem safe, but inflammation-causing ingredients and toxic chemicals may be lurking in your favorite products. To maintain your skin's optimal health, you should avoid any skincare product or treatment that causes inflammation, skin damage, or increases your risk of disease. In this chapter, we have investigated the most popular cosmetic ingredients and separated the good from the bad.

- Alpha hydroxy acids exfoliate the skin and cause inflammation. But not all AHAs are the same: Glycolic acid damages the epidermis, while lactic acid and mandelic acid can benefit the skin if used in moderation.
- Retinoic acid, a popular prescription, also inflames the skin, interferes with the skin's normal turnover and repair process, and compromises the epidermis. Also avoid the oral form of retinoic acid, Accutane, which is frequently used for acne.
- Hydroquinone is used to treat hyperpigmentation but poses some cancer risks, can be toxic to certain organs, and ages the skin.
- Steroids are prescribed to control inflammation but can lead to trauma, atrophy, and scarring.
- Antibiotics are also commonly prescribed to treat rosacea and acne but their use can compromise your digestive and immune systems.
- Some common beauty ingredients, like vitamin K and caffeine, sound healthy and are even found in the foods we eat, but you should also steer clear of them.
- Vitamin C is another example of how a good thing can go bad. It causes inflammation and increases free radicals but can be safe to use in lower concentrations and dry powder form.
- Peptides are safe as long as they are used with ingredients that correct damage.
- Sodium lauryl sulfate is found in face washes and liquid soaps, but studies find that it's an irritant.
- Parabens, including methylparaben, propylparaben, and butylparaben, are chemical preservatives that researchers have discovered in breast tumors.
- Ceramides claim to moisturize dry skin but may actually promote aging.
- Glycols (propylene glycol, ethylene glycol, and polyethylene glycol, or PEG) strip lipids, increase free radicals, and cause dehydration.
- Topical oxygen therapy appears to be effective, but this treatment generates free radicals in the epidermis.

Part 3

~

Dr. Johnson's Plan for Youthful, Healthy Skin

CHAPTER FIVE

The Basic Plan: Work with the Skin

~

The dermis thins at a rate of 1 percent per year
after the age of 30. The epidermis, by contrast,
does not thin at all during our entire lifespan.

~

THE GOAL OF HEALTHY skincare is to assist the skin in executing its basic functions. As the largest organ in the human body, the skin is exquisitely designed to regulate and manage its daily conditions and responses to internal and external factors. The guiding principle is simple: Work with the skin. Most of us, to the extent that we support our skin in fulfilling its duties, tend to enjoy a clear and healthful complexion most of the time.

That said, there are times when the skin will erupt and present conditions that are, to put it bluntly, undesirable. At such times, intervention may be the most appropriate course. Pain, itching, discomfort, and embarrassment are all perfectly valid reasons to seek help, whether through the services of a physician or a skincare professional, or through over-the-counter products and home remedies. It is critical that we understand and appreciate, however, what the skin is doing at such times, and why.

Before we subject ourselves to daily exfoliation routines or slather on the acids, it's valuable to recognize that the skin operates on a natural cycle of exfoliation. It's also important to understand that the stratum corneum—or the outermost layer of the epidermis—is comprised largely of "dead" skin cells. Yet these dead cells serve a purpose. The very layer we seek to remove by exfoliating or applying acid treatments is an effective filter that protects the dermis from UV radiation, environmental toxins, and dehydration.

Remember this fact: The dermis thins at a rate of 1 percent per year beginning in our 20s. The epidermis, by contrast, does not thin at all during our entire lifespan. Keep this in mind when evaluating dermatological treatments and therapies. While the epidermis measures a mere .33 millimeters in thickness, it bears enormous responsibility to prevent against infection and fluid loss. Were the epidermis to thin at the same rate that the dermis thins, not a single one of us would live past the age of 50. A chronically thinning epidermis would result in lethal levels of infection and dehydration.

There is not a physician in the world who would recommend exfoliating the skin of a child. We know that the child's skin is functioning optimally—and yet it functions exactly the same way the skin functions in a healthy adult. A healthy 10-year-old has roughly a 30-day exfoliation cycle, which is the same for healthy adult skin. And yet, we have decided in the last 30 years that this remarkable organ, this 24/7 extraordinarily hard-working machine, doesn't know what it is doing. The entire skincare industry has made forced exfoliation the gold standard. Is that based on science? Was there ever a research study that showed the dermal benefits to removing the surface of the skin? Absolutely not. This entire strategy has been based on confusing visible evidence.

Before we analyze the benefits and harmful effects of exfoliation, let us remember that the epidermis slows down because it has to. The declining level of nutrients that occurs in everyone's skin forces the epidermis to slow down in order to be able to maintain a complete barrier. The result is that the outermost layers of skin appear old or ragged. The truth of the matter is that our epidermis does become old.

Or, to use a more apt term, our stratum corneum becomes stale. As the exfoliation cycle slows, we hold on to damaged or dead skin for longer periods of time.

Beginning some time in our 30s, many of us begin to feel a rising pressure to maintain (or return to) a youthful look for our skin. For some reason between the ages of 10 and 30, we supposedly transform from people who need no exfoliation to people who, for various reasons, must undertake exfoliation as part of our daily regimen. But is that really the case? Must we truly intervene daily in our skin's natural processes?

~

I view unnecessary exfoliation as an assault on the skin.

~

For the majority of us, the answer to these questions is no. The body has already placed terrific priority on the health of the epidermis. This is evidenced by the fact that, despite thinning of the dermis and other symptoms of aging, the epidermis remains, by and large, intact throughout our lifetimes. This is why I view unnecessary exfoliation as an assault on the skin. This attack triggers an "emergency repair response," which is the only reason why the skin speeds up its renewal rate. Many people have proposed that exfoliation makes the skin healthier, so that's why the skin speeds up. But the scientific evidence refutes that. Instead, we have seen rates of skin cancer, rosacea, melasma, and more conditions soar in the last few decades.

While I understand the desire to preserve the skin's youthful appearance, you have to wonder just how we got here. The only scientific evidence on exfoliation shows it increases damage, speeds aging, and increases cancer risk. Rather than force the skin to exfoliate before it is ready to—and thus force nutrients up to the epidermis—our approach should be to feed and nourish the dermis. Remember that the epidermis exists to protect the dermis. Think of it as a "wearguard." Rather than focus on the wearguard, we ought to invest our efforts in the part of the skin that is really aging. When that underlying tissue is healthy, our faces will reveal the youthful appeal we're so eager to achieve.

Never Add Inflammation

If the guiding principle of healthy skincare is to work with the skin, then the most important rule is this: *Don't add inflammation.* We've already seen how exfoliation leads to an increase in free radicals, and we've established that, without proper balance, free radicals are bad. The best way to avoid free radicals is to avoid irritation and anything that increases UV exposure.

Exfoliation, of course, is a natural, daily event of the skin. The difference between what the skin does on its own and our forced exfoliation strategies is significant. The skin only releases the top layer of the stratum corneum when the bottom layers of the epidermis complete its replacement layer. Essentially, the skin pushes off the top layer by adding to the "stack of dead cells" first. In this way, the barrier is constantly intact. Forced exfoliation tears down protection without regard for what the rest of the epidermis is doing, which is why it is so inflammatory.

Exfoliation for exfoliation's sake is a travesty of modern skincare practice. However, when exfoliation is the result of efforts to rejuvenate the dermis, then there is a justification for it. The key is to find procedures that actually rebuild dermal collagen thickness. To this end, I can appreciate a mild, monthly exfoliation—for example, in order to deliver liposomal nutrients (see sidebar, "Liposomal Delivery," on page 80) more effectively to the dermis without leaving particles trapped in the epidermis. In such cases there is a clear and measurable net benefit to the exfoliation undertaken. But for the purpose of lightening the appearance of pigment or plumping surrounding tissues, exfoliation widely misses the mark as any kind of skincare solution.

Restore the Barrier

Healthy skin relies on a healthy epidermis. We've talked about the epidermis as the wearguard that protects the dermis. I've cautioned that, while it's important to maintain a healthy dermis, we cannot afford to do

Exfoliation actually upsets the atomic makeup
of our skin, loosing a fury of free radicals
that run around seeking stability
and causing chain reactions at the atomic level.
This eventually take a toll
on the cellular makeup of the skin.

so at the expense of the epidermis. Yet, this is exactly what happens when we strip away the normal functioning layers of the epidermis in an effort to reach and rejuvenate the deeper skin layers. We really must respect and protect the natural function of the epidermis as a healthy barrier between the dermis and the open air.

One easy way to protect the epidermis is to dial down the temperature on your water heater and shorten the amount of time you spend bathing. Excess heat not only creates inflammation in your skin, but combined with the chlorine that is added to municipal water supplies and the soaps we use to complete our bathing ritual, long, hot showers and long soaks in the tub alter our skin's natural pH balance. Exposure to heat and chlorine also strips away our skin's lipids—naturally occurring fatty molecules that store energy and help protect the skin from the elements. This increases the production of free radicals.

Meanwhile, too many soaps, body washes, astringents, toners, and lotions are overly aggressive in their pursuit of cleanliness. Alcohol in small doses—less than 5 percent—is not necessarily a bad thing, but alcohol-heavy products strip away lipids and actively inflame the skin. So too, does sodium lauryl sulfate, a chemical commonly found in soaps and detergents for the express purpose of creating lather. While we may associate this rich lather with effectiveness, it actually does more harm than good. Thanks to its efficacy as a stripping agent, sodium lauryl sulfate is a chief ingredient in such industrial cleaning supplies as engine degreasers and floor-buffing solutions. Is that really what you want on your skin? It is even used in dermatologic research

ent that inflames the skin whenever they are testing topi-
ammatories.

.mericans are admirably devoted to hygiene, we're actually
clea.   to the detriment of our skin. It's better to have a little bit of
dirt on your skin than to overcleanse and remove the protective lipids.
The free radicals that come from dirt and particles lodged in the natural oils on our skin are minor compared to the flood of free radicals
released when we start stripping away the epidermal layers and their
lipid cohorts.

Penetrate the Appropriate Target

By now, some readers may be wondering about effective topical nutrition—and rightfully so, especially with all the talk about free radicals.
If free radicals cause oxidation, can't we counteract the effects of that
process by introducing antioxidants to the skin? And doesn't it make
sense to do so topically, since the skin's surface is where free radicals
wreak their havoc? To answer these questions, let's examine how topical
supplements work, and then we'll have a better sense of why they can
come up short.

While many of the minerals and vitamins featured in the ingredients
lists of any number of top-selling supplements are beneficial to the skin,
topical methods of delivery almost certainly fail to render the prom-
ised improvements. This is because the vast majority of the ingredients
of any lotion, cream, or ointment become trapped in the epidermis
(which is designed to act as a filter, after all) and never reach their target
in the dermis. In other words, it's nearly impossible to nourish the dermis from the outside in without a great delivery system. The issue is not
just lack of efficacy. When vitamins and minerals get stuck in the skin,
they often become a source of inflammation, so, unfortunately, more is
not better.

Consider the example of vitamin C (preferably "L-ascorbic acid"),
which we know is good for the skin. At lower compositions—ideally
around 6 to 10 percent (depending on skin sensitivity)—vitamin C can
nourish and support the skin. There is a common belief among skincare practitioners, however, that vitamin C at 20 percent composition

~

*It's much better to have a little bit of dirt
on your skin than to over-cleanse
and remove the protective lipids.*

≈

will maximize the amount of the nutrient your skin can store in order to maintain healthful vitamin C levels for up to several days. Generally speaking, however, we have no need to store excess vitamin C for several days because it's not hard to replenish it on a daily basis. Moreover, we can also supplement skin levels *internally* without relying on topical applications of the nutrient, especially since topical vitamin C only boasts a 2 percent penetration rate. That low penetration rate means that the bulk of the vitamin gets lodged in the epidermis and never reaches its target. No matter how healthful the nutrient is to the dermis, when caught in the epidermis the same particles can be interpreted as irritants and actually incite inflammation as they oxidize and force exfoliation. This leads to tissue problems in the long run.

The same is true with other antioxidants. While research has proven that antioxidants are effective at arresting skin aging, we run into delivery problems when attempting to apply antioxidants topically because their size often prevents absorption. Unfortunately, only a small percentage of the applied ingredients penetrate the surface of the skin. As with vitamin C, it may be necessary to introduce antioxidants internally and allow the body to process and distribute additional antioxidants to the dermis and epidermis from the inside out. It may also be similarly efficacious to add the components needed to make antioxidants.

I'm no enemy of convenience, but when taking our health into consideration, convenience must yield to efficacy. It would be a beautiful thing if we could wake up every day and spread antioxidants on our faces to battle free radicals and keep us looking youthful. Indeed, many of us attempt to do exactly that. But the topical delivery of antioxidants and other supplements routinely fails to achieve meaningful success. Of more concern, it can lead to greater damage due to the

ɔmal Delivery

A liposome is a minute sphere made of various materials that are designed to either make ingredients mix better in solution, or more commonly, to enhance penetration through the epidermis. The material I prefer—and the one backed by the best research—is phosphatidylcholine. The reason it works so well is because it is identical to the material that composes our cell membranes. Over the years, scientists have devised ways to engineer liposomes for the express purpose of delivering drugs to affected areas of the body to fight disease. Thanks to the nature of the liposome itself, molecules that make up the liposome's membrane communicate naturally with molecules of a cell membrane. Once this bonding occurs, the contents of the liposome react upon the cell. In this way, liposomal drug delivery has been particularly effective in battling cancer, because chemicals or drugs can be directed at the site of a tumor to attack cancerous cells or boost healthy cells before cancer has a chance to erode them.

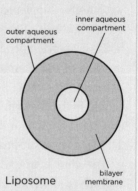

outer aqueous compartment

inner aqueous compartment

bilayer membrane

Liposome

In skin care, liposomal delivery of antioxidants, vitamins, nutrients, and other ingredients has obvious advantages to normal topical delivery methods. Liposomal ingredients can be ingested in capsule form or applied through the surface of the skin. Thanks to the lipid-loving nature of the liposome's outer membrane, whatever is contained within the liposome will be absorbed by the cells once it reaches the appropriate target cells. The liposome bonds with these cells, thus delivering the cargo contained inside the tiny bubble. Furthermore, liposomal engineering and liposome preparation methods can result in vesicles designed to deliver their payloads to specific cells, depending on variances such as pH or charge. Thus a burst of antioxidants, taken internally, can be preserved until they reach the appropriate levels of the dermis and epidermis to do the most good.

It's nearly impossible to nourish the dermis from the outside in without a great delivery system.

entrapment of particles in the epidermis. The best way to boost antioxidant levels in the skin is through healthy nutrition, which compels the body to produce its own antioxidants based on cellular reactions occurring in balance with the body's unique set of needs. This needs to be followed by using topical agents that work with these larger-sized antioxidants, including mineral cofactors like zinc, copper, and selenium, but also ingredients that increase circulation like niacinamide and 1,3 beta glucan.

Increase Skin Nutrition

As we work with the skin to promote health throughout the organ, we must attend to the functions we hope to improve. For example, we want to increase dermal nutrition through vasodilation, thus boosting immune activity and providing nourishment to the dermis. When we target the dermis, we want to increase the number of fibroblasts available, and we want to improve their activity. We also want to increase the number of macrophages to improve the health of the immune system relative to the dermis. To improve skin nutrition, we need to increase the number of antioxidants and amino acids that effectively reach their targets, and increase mineral cofactors to speed enzymatic processes and boost the metabolism.

Another component of good skin nutrition, believe it or not, is the sun. Just as plants enjoy the benefits of balanced sun exposure, so, too, do humans. Our skin is designed to accept energy from the sun, and we need the vitamin D that the sun's rays impart. Our skin naturally possesses and produces the amino acids, antioxidants, and cofactors to tolerate a certain amount of direct sunlight every day. In fact, the skin is naturally engineered to take anywhere from five to 60 minutes of sunlight daily (depending on the individual) without the risk of incurring long-term damage. This is not to say that damage does not occur, but rather that the level of inflammation created is handled well by the skin's repair processes.

While we must recognize the risks of too much sun exposure, it is also a mistake to overprotect against the sun. To this end, if you want to boost nutrients to the skin, aim to get 15 minutes a day of direct sunlight exposure without cosmetics or sunscreens impeding absorption. Consider maximizing the potential benefit of these 15 minutes by exposing your upper torso, not just your hands and face, without increasing any risk of damage. This "sun time" should ideally occur in the morning or late-afternoon hours when less damage is inflicted by UVB rays.

~

Another component of good skin nutrition,
believe it or not, is the sun.

∾

Collagen Breakdown and Healthy Skin

Many of us think that collagen breakdown is a good thing, but the reality is very different. The only reason our skin breaks down collagen is because the collagen is damaged and must be disposed of. The skin quickly identifies bad, or damaged, collagen, and it knows when and how to rapidly digest this collagen while preserving the surrounding tissues. In that sense, collagen breakdown is a good thing because it disposes of unhealthy matter. Remember, damaged collagen collapses, making the skin appear even older. But if we stop at that conclusion, we'll never understand why our collagen is damaged in the first place. This, I believe, is the danger in assuming that beauty is skin deep. In order to stall skin breakdown (aging), we have to stall collagen breakdown through prevention. In other words, we've got to stop collagen damage before it starts. Healthy nutrition can help. So can avoiding inflammation. Retinoic acid is popular for its purported antiaging properties, but here we see a major disconnect: Retinoic acid increases damage to collagen by affecting the epidermal barrier. Then it reduces the skin's ability to fix that collagen. This likely explains the main reason why retinoic acid has been such a disappointment.

Take another naturally occurring substance, ceramides, which are lipids the skin produces to protect its outer layers. Generally, ceramides are a good thing, so it's not outrageous that skincare manufacturers have seized upon them to promote skin products. But ceramides figure into the skin's secondary feedback loop. If you add a ceramide moisturizer to the epidermis, the skin registers those additional ceramides and *slows down the epidermal turnover rate* specifically in response to a confusing signal from their introduction into the skin. The resulting artificially slowed exfoliation cycle likely only adds to the frustration with the skin's function and appearance rather than protecting and rejuvenating the skin, as so much marketing propaganda will promise.

Instead of adding retinoic acid or ceramides to the skin, we should use ingredients along the lines of retinaldehyde in our skincare products. Retinaldehyde prompts the skin to begin a chemical conversion to create its own retinoic acid. The skin only modifes what it needs of the retinaldehyde molecules, which prevents it from becoming irritated or damaged by excess retinoic acid. What it doesn't need, it stores so that an integrated balance of naturally occurring chemicals can work in harmony in the skin. Compare this to slathering on a dollop of Retin-A® cream. Only a small percentage of the critical ingredients ever reach the target areas of the dermis. The rest build up in the epidermis, creating fodder for oxidation and skin irritation.

To Sum It Up

The skin is an ingeniously devised system of sensors, barriers, tissues, and cells, all of which work in harmony—when we let them—with the other systems of the body to protect us as we age. Any truly natural approach to skincare must work with the skin. It must understand how the skin is designed to function and assist the skin during times of trouble rather than intervene or work against the skin's innate responses.

rt we make to interrupt a skin function must take into account
ted functions that will also be delayed or interrupted.

In order to help the skin achieve the balance it seeks, any treatment
we use must avoid creating inflammation. I cannot stress this enough. It
seems simple, but once we investigate the raft of products and procedures
on the market, we realize that the bulk of them result in inflammation.
In the rare instance that the inflammation is mild and there are benefits
to the long-term health of the skin, then such infrequent treatment (no
more than monthly) may be explored.

While working with the skin and avoiding inflammation, it's also
important to understand how we can maintain and restore the dermis and epidermis to their most effective levels of health. Long, hot
showers and application of overaggressive soaps are pervasive causes
of damage to the skin. The heat, chlorine, and stripping agents combine to remove all of the lipids from our skin. But we need some of
those lipids in order to protect the dermis. A little dirt is essential to
healthy skin.

As we maintain and improve our skin, it's critical to focus internally
rather than externally to achieve results. The topical application of minerals, vitamins, and supplements generally delivers only a fraction of the
necessary quantity of key ingredients to the dermis. In other words, most
of your creams, lotions, toners, and moisturizers end up trapped in the
epidermis. Once there, those same ingredients that promise to improve
your skin can actually cause more harm than good. Instead, turn to the
natural resources found in a healthy diet, get appropriate sun exposure,
and ingest supplements as needed to help the skin right any imbalances
you may experience from time to time.

Finally, remember that the skin is smart. When we introduce too
much of a good thing, such as ceramides or retinoic acid, the skin actually reads the reactions taking place at the epidermal level and changes
its normal behavior. In other words, we need to focus more energy on
providing the skin with the ingredients it needs daily and less time sec-
ond-guessing the skin's abilities to manage itself.

Don't be fooled by fads or instant solutions. Work with your skin
from the inside out and take the long view on where you want your skin

to be in a few decades. Remember that most improvements from our current approach to skincare are nothing more than trauma induced— temporary responses by the skin that do more harm than good. Real repair takes more time. As you observe the degeneration of your skin, it's natural to want to take steps to slow or stop the process. The skincare industry has built its fortune on that exact response, but don't be fooled. The likelihood of achieving the skin you desire and the appearance that makes you happy increases as you take time to work with your skin and treat all the systems of the body harmoniously.

CHAPTER SIX

Healthy Skin from the Inside Out: Nutrition, the Digestive Tract, and Our Skin

THE BODY IS A remarkable, fully integrated system. What happens in one part of the body affects what happens elsewhere, so it should come as no surprise that our internal health has everything to do with the health of our skin. Our skin relies on the nourishment in our diets for much of the sustenance—vitamins, minerals, antioxidants, lipids, and hydration—it needs to survive and thrive.

But a healthy diet is only the beginning of the story. We also need our digestive system to function properly in order to optimally digest and utilize the food that we eat. A compromised digestive tract can actually cause or amplify our skin's problems, even when our diet is balanced.

Unfortunately, the typical Western diet fails us in two ways: It does not provide the nutrition our bodies need, and it taxes our digestive tract to the point that it is incapable of properly performing its necessary functions. The net effect is a significant decline in nutrients that are absorbed from our food, as well as poorly digested food lingering in our system. When food is not properly broken down within the stomach, it becomes a source of irritation, allergies, and inflammation as it passes through the digestive tract. Our bodies are designed to handle a lot of assaults—large

> The ill-conceived Western diet is the
> main reason for disease in our society—and that
> includes skin diseases.

hits of toxins and a variety of adverse situations—but they are not resilient enough to cope with the constant bombardment of food-related toxins. Our diets are slowly but surely damaging the entire digestive system and, in the process, we are triggering an increase in immune activity and tissue damage throughout the body. History and research have been very clear on this matter: The ill-conceived Western diet is the main reason for disease in our society—and that includes skin disease.

The good news is that our diets are entirely within our control. We can choose what and how much we eat. And armed with information on how the body uses food and what specific foods it needs to function at its best, we can make the healthiest choices possible.

Digestion 101: Anatomy and Function of the Digestive Tract

The digestive tract is the path food travels as it makes its way through the body, beginning at the mouth and ending at the anus (with the esophagus, stomach, small intestine, and large intestine in between). The mouth, stomach, and small intestine all contain tiny glands that secrete enzymes to help digest food. Additional fluids, acids, and enzymes are supplied by the pancreas and the liver.

When we eat, the body breaks the food it into small molecules of nutrients that can be absorbed into the blood and delivered to the cells. Digestion begins in the mouth and is essentially completed in the small intestine.

As we chew our food, we break apart some of its chemical compounds and absorb nutrients through the tissues in our mouth—what is called our buccal mucosa. That allows the body to recognize and identify the nutrients, and prepare the rest of the digestive tract to

Chew Chew

As we've learned, digestion begins in the mouth. Unfortunately, many of us tend to underestimate the importance of the very first step in the digestive process: chewing. Our strong teeth are designed to begin the breakdown of food. But many of us are in such a rush to eat that we swallow our food without properly chewing it first. Ideally we should chew each bite of food 20 to 25 times before swallowing. The next time you're eating, keep track of how many times you chew each bite. I'll bet you'll find that you chew only five to 10 times at most.

The result of our poor chewing habits is twofold. First, the stomach has to work harder and longer to digest large pieces of food since these haven't been broken down adequately by the enzymes in the mouth. Second, the stomach hasn't had enough time to prepare adequately for the food's arrival—meaning it may not have the acids and/or enzymes on hand to digest the food properly.

The first—and easiest—step you can take to improve your digestion is to slow down and chew each bite 20 to 25 times before swallowing.

process and assimilate them. Depending on the type of food we are eating, the body reacts in a specific way. When the body senses that it is being fed protein, it increases stomach acid and enzyme production so that the small intestine can break the protein into the amino acids it needs. These amino acids will then be used to build cells, muscular tissue, skin tissue, hair, and just about everything in between. Proteins need a more acidic environment for digestion than do carbohydrates, so the body accommodates.

When we start chewing a piece of steak, our body signals the stomach to increase its acid levels and lets the pancreas know that it needs to secrete specific enzymes (trypsin and chymotyrypsin) into the small bowel to finish the job of breaking down the proteins. The mouth recognizes reacts by reducing amylase and other enzymes that are not appropriate for protein digestion. The steak travels down the esophagus to the stomach, where the acid environment breaks down

Amino Acid Supplements

Amino acids are not designed to handle the high-acid environment of the stomach, which is why complex proteins—which take more time to break down into amino acids—are more usable for the body. For that reason, amino acid supplements, which enter the stomach already in their individual form, should be taken with some sort of a bicarbonate solution to protect them from excessive acid damage.

the protein enough to release small peptides and amino acids into the small bowel.

Now that the proteins have gone through significant digestion, the stomach begins to move the broken-down protein components toward the small bowel, where they are more protected in an alkaline environment. The body knows it needs a high-acid environment in the stomach in order to break that steak down into usable amino acids. It also knows it needs the alkaline environment of the small bowel for the individual nutrients to be protected, further digested, and absorbed.

Once foods make it to the small bowel, amino acids and minerals are absorbed into the bloodstream. The small bowel is remarkable; it has a length of about 15 feet, but if it were to be fully stretched out it actually is as large as a tennis court. That is our key to maximizing absorption. The small bowel absorbs about 90 percent of the fluid and foods we take in. The bulk of the remaining food debris, including some potentially valuable dietary nutrients, then works its way to the large intestine, where our good bacteria scavenge for more nutrients and absorb fluids (including the digestive juices that we've used thus far) to keep our bodies hydrated. The unused food continues through the body and is eliminated as waste.

When we eat carbohydrates, the body reacts differently than it does to protein. The enzyme amylase, which exists in our saliva, begins the process of carbohydrate breakdown. That's why it's a good idea whenever you are eating carbohydrates (e.g., bread, potatoes, sugar, pasta) to pay special attention to chewing your food thoroughly. Carbohydrates need a more alkaline environment than proteins do, so the stomach does not release as much acid in preparation for carbohydrate digestion. As carbohydrates are broken down, the sugar molecules are managed within the small bowel, where they're absorbed into the system.

~

I believe that a number of chronic conditions—
including constipation, diarrhea, acid reflux,
and a variety of skin conditions—can all
be traced back to improper food combining and
the effects it and our otherwise toxic foods have
on the digestive lining and juices involved.

~

Food Combining

Since the body creates different environments for different food groups, we enter confusing territory when we combine foods. It makes sense from an evolutionary perspective; back in our hunter-gatherer days, we would come across a fruit tree and likely eat that fruit as our meal. Later on, we might kill an animal and have meat for that meal, but very rarely did we have meat and fruit in the same sitting.

I contend (along with many other nutritional experts) that our bodies still benefit from segmented eating. In the case of steak, I would recommend eating it alone or only with other foods that require a high-acid environment to break down. In fact, I advise against eating anything that might send a conflicting signal to the digestive tract (potatoes, for instance) for an hour before or after eating the steak. Otherwise, the digestive system is being told by the bite of steak that we need high acid production in order to break that steak down, and then it is getting a second message that we need a low acid environment to digest the potatoes. The result? The steak is not properly digested because the stomach is not acidic enough, and the potatoes become damaged because the stomach is too acidic. The net effect of this is that toxic and inflammatory events en within our digestive tract and we don't absorb as many nutrients from our food as we should.

I believe that a number of chronic conditions—including constipation, diarrhea, acid reflux, and a variety of skin conditions—can all be traced back to improper food combining and the effects it and otherwise toxic foods have on the digestive lining and juices involved. Add to this the struggles adults have digesting dairy products and we can see why most Americans suffer some kind of digestive disturbance at some time in their life.

Addicted to Inflammation: Why Does Eating Bad Feel So Good?

Of course, it's not just our digestive tract that reacts to the foods we eat (and how and when we eat them). The entire body is affected by our nutrition, or lack thereof. A huge problem with the foods we eat is that many of them are inflammatory. Some of the main offenders are white flour, hydrogenated fats, refined sugar, artificial additives, preservatives, sodium benzoate, sulfites, nitrites, and pesticides. Unfortunately, these components can be found in a significant portion of the typical Western diet.

When our body senses that we've ingested something toxic or inflammatory to the system, it releases cortisol and beta-endorphins. Now cortisol and beta-endorphins are both feel-good chemicals, so when we eat foods that are bad for us we actually get a momentary high. It's that high that leads us, ultimately, to become addicted to unhealthy foods. In fact, recent research found that certain foods trigger a chemical response in the brain very similar to the response

Where Do Those Toxins Go?

Cortisol tends to promote the accumulation of toxins within the belly. In women, we can also see the accumulation of toxins in the outside of the thighs and buttocks. However, different individuals store their fat and toxins in different parts of the body.

Because of our farming practices, environmental pollution, and overconsumption, the foods we produce in this country don't contain the vitamins and minerals needed to prevent malnourishment and disease.

created by cocaine. I believe it's our addiction to inflammatory foods that has caused America's overwhelming problem with obesity and inflammatory health conditions.

When inflammatory foods—particularly sugar—enter the system, the pancreas releases insulin, which drives sugar into the cells so it can be used as energy. The release of insulin, along with cortisol and beta-endorphins, is actually designed to put out the fires caused by all the free-floating glucose that can damage blood vessel walls and create inflammatory reactions within other tissues.

Case in point: emotional overeating. When people are feeling down and depressed, many of them turn to unhealthy foods. Why? Is it because a full stomach boosts mood? No, it's because subconsciously we know that inflammatory foods will cause our bodies to release the bolus of feel-good hormones. Unfortunately, the hormone effects are very brief. No sooner do we throw out the wrapper from our fast-food meal then the effects start to wear off. So then what do we do? We find something else to eat—a box of candy, perhaps—that will keep the high going.

It's my personal opinion that this country as a whole is suffering from several different medical ailments that all center on the damage food causes. The toxicity from these unhealthy foods leads to the high levels of cortisol. This then causes a decline in the body's ability to repair the tissues because the excess overwhelms our system. If you were to eat one M&M every 10 minutes over several hours, your body would experience much less inflammation and aging than if you were to eat the entire bag in five minutes. Why? Because the body is able to respond to each M&M

appropriately. It will create an alkaline environment to break the candy down so that the glucose doesn't become damaged. (Glucose on its own can be quite damaging in excess, but acid-damaged glucose causes a much more inflammatory response in the system.)

Your body will put out insulin to try to store the sugar for later use, but it takes a while for the insulin to drive the glucose into the cell. So, if you were to eat the M&Ms quickly, the glucose would float freely within the bloodstream while the body tried to accommodate it. Of course, too much glucose in the bloodstream is toxic and causes inflammation in a lot of different areas, leading to a release of cortisol. This slows down the repair process, leads to damaged blood vessel walls, and even causes atherosclerosis. In the case of diabetes, many of the small blood vessels actually can close from the amount of damage that is created. What's more, cortisol has an effect on all of our tissues, including the skin, so every time we eat a box of candy, we ultimately are creating an aging event in our skin.

Lack of Nutrition in Foods

In addition to being highly inflammatory, the typical American diet has another problem: It's lacking in nutrition. Because of our farming practices, environmental pollution, and overconsumption, the foods we produce in this country often do not contain the vitamins and minerals needed to prevent malnourishment and disease.

Fish is a perfect illustration of how our shortsightedness harms our food supply. How sad a state is it that we must be warned against eating too much fish—a perfectly healthy source of protein, vitamins, minerals, and essential fatty acids—because our oceans and rivers have become so polluted? Instead we are encouraged to eat "safe" farm-raised fish. But these fish don't contain the same level of nutrition because they are not eating the varied diet they would normally get in the wild. There is nothing sadder to me than buying salmon, only to read on the label that there is artificial color added because of nutritional deficiencies.

This nutritional shortage is also found in most fruits and vegetables due to our overused farmlands. Because of current agricultural practices, the fields our food comes from are now mineral deficient. Of course, the

Where Do Those Toxins Go?

Cortisol tends to promote the accumulation of toxins within the belly. In women, we can also see the accumulation of toxins in the outside of the thighs and buttocks. However, different individuals store their fat and toxins in different parts of the body.

Eating carbohydrates and protein together confuses the digestive system by sending mixed signals about whether we need an acidic or alkaline environment. For that reason, I recommend waiting one hour between eating from those different food groups.

Our bodies are not designed to receive a great deal of hydration while we are eating, because it can interfere with the important work of the digestive juices produced within the digestive tract.

ideal way for us to get our vitamins and minerals is through these foods, yet more and more, we are forced to turn to (less nourishing) supplementation to make up for this vital nutritional support.

8 Steps to Optimal Nutrition

Even in light of our lackluster American diet, we do have options about what and how we eat. We can maximize both our nutritional intake and our body's ability to digest the food we eat by following these eight important dietary rules:

- **START OFF EASY.** A digestive system that has long been mistreated needs some TLC to get back on track. Since most of us start off with a digestive tract that has been abused since a very early age, some recovery is needed. When you first start to overhaul your diet, include easily digestible foods that will allow you to optimize your nutritional intake. A great way to do this is by juicing fruits and vegetables. This begins the breakdown process before the food even enters the body. By giving your body easily digestible food for a period of several months, you'll see a recovery in the digestive lining that, in time, allows you to eat normal foods.

~

Our bodies function better when they are not exposed
to processed foods like bleached flour, refined sugars,
preservatives, alcohol, and hydrogenated fats.

~

- **EAT LOCALLY.** Because we've strayed so far from local eating, our foods contain preservatives to allow for longer shipping and shelf life. In addition, foods have lost much of their nutritional value simply by virtue of being processed for preservation. As soon as a fruit or vegetable is harvested, or removed from its natural habitat, it immediately begins to lose nutrients and oxidize. This is why choosing fresh, locally grown produce is so important. What's more, fruits and vegetables from farms within your region are more likely to meet your specific mineral needs than those grown far away.

- **EAT ORGANICALLY.** In order to avoid the toxic pesticides and hormones present in conventionally grown foods, eat organic food whenever possible. This is especially important when it comes to dairy and meat, which often contain antibiotics and hormones if they have been raised conventionally.

- **INCLUDE WHOLE GRAINS.** The body digests whole grains slowly. This is advantageous because it helps to prevent a spike in blood sugar. Remember that M&Ms example? That applies to the grains we eat, too. If we eat refined grains, we create an inflammatory reaction in our system because the grain has been modified and is less recognizable to our small intestine. But if we eat a whole grain, the time it takes to break down that carbohydrate source gives the body time to assimilate it more appropriately.

- **SUPPLEMENT WITH MINERALS.** The absolute best way to get the minerals your body needs is through vegetables and fruits. Unfortunately, conventional farming techniques have depleted the soil (and the veggies that grow in it) of its minerals. Unless you know the farmland where your vegetables are grown and are confident in the health of the soil, it's a good idea to supplement.

Nutrition Lessons From a Dentist

Weston A. Price, DDS, (1870–1948) was a dentist from Cleveland who traveled the world studying isolated, non-industrialized peoples. During his travels, he searched for the causes of dental decay and physical degeneration. What he found was that isolated peoples who ate unadulterated, traditional diets had healthy, straight, cavity-free teeth and strong bodies. The "Westernized" societies he studied, on the other hand, suffered widespread dental decay and physical problems. He looked to the staples of the industrialized diet as the reason for this disease: sugar, white flour, alcohol, pasteurized milk, and preservative-laden food.

Traditional diets, however, focus on whole foods and provide four times the calcium and other minerals, and 10 times the fat-soluble vitamins from animal foods. When non-industrialized societies were introduced to the "civilized" diets, the effect was striking: Suddenly problems like high blood pressure, obesity, and dental crowding, which had never occurred before in these populations, were rampant.

What we can learn from these observations is that our bodies function better when they are not exposed to processed foods like bleached flour, refined sugars, preservatives, alcohol, and hydrogenated fats.

- **GOOD FATS.** Many people are afraid of fats. They won't eat anything with oil or fat in it because they are concerned about cholesterol and other related problems. But, in many cases, oils and fats can be quite healthy. The body needs lipids, especially omega-3 and omega-9 fatty acids. We know from history that getting omegas through sources like cold-pressed olive oil and other oils is beneficial and does not promote disease. Other good sources of these healthy fats include fish, avocados, nuts, and seeds.
- **CAREFUL COMBINING.** As I explained earlier, eating carbohydrates and protein together confuses the digestive system by sending mixed signals about whether it should create an acidic or alkaline

ronment. For that reason, I recommend waiting one hour between
ng from those different food groups.

- **HYDRATE, BUT AT THE RIGHT TIME.** While hydration is absolutely necessary for survival and health—research shows it improves metabolism, detoxification, circulation, and oxygenation—we need to be careful about when we hydrate. Our bodies are not designed to receive a great deal of hydration while we are eating because it can interfere with the important work of the digestive juices. When we eat, we should minimize how much we drink and wait an hour after eating before hydrating significantly.

Topical Nutrition

The food we eat is but one source of nutrition for our skin. Another way we can deliver nutrients to the epidermis and dermis is topically—which is one reason the skincare industry thrives. But, as we've learned, the process of delivering nutrients via the epidermis is tricky. While the epidermis benefits from certain minerals like copper, zinc, selenium, and magnesium, excess levels can be inflammatory and can cause problems within the skin. The same is true of vitamins A, B, C, and E, all of which—as we've seen—can become trapped in the epidermis. So, even though these nutrients are beneficial to the dermis, they are rarely delivered adequately to that portion of the skin. I believe that with any type of skin-nutrition program, the delivery mechanism needs to be through liposomes. Liposomal delivery entails encasing the nutrient in a lipid sac that protects it and allows it to penetrate more deeply into the dermis. While this still doesn't ensure perfect delivery, liposomes can increase penetration up to 1,000 percent.

With that in mind, there are certain specific vitamins, minerals, antioxidants, and other nutrients that I recommend for the skin.

VITAMIN A

Vitamin A is an important nutrient that should be supplemented both internally and topically, but the type of vitamin A you choose is very important. The scientific evidence clearly points us in the direction of one specific type: retinaldehyde. I know retinaldehyde sounds like formaldehyde, which leads some people to think it's bad for them. But the "aldehyde" simply describes part of the vitamin's chemical nature—not any level of toxicity. In fact, retinaldehyde is found in most of our fat cells, since this is where the body stores it. I think it is the preferred form of vitamin A because the other types of the nutrient (other than Retin-A®) are 1,000 times weaker than retinaldehyde. Only Retin-A® and retinaldehyde have enough collagen-stimulating activity to have a significant impact on the dermis. In fact, retinaldehyde has many of the same effects on UV-induced sun damage as does Retin-A®, including repairing elastic fibers and collagen. The advantage of retinaldehyde over Retin-A® is that retinaldehyde is both nontoxic and is stored by the body.

In the scientific lierature, retinaldehyde has proven to be as strong as Retin-A® and non-irritating, so it clearly has an advantage in the vitamin A category. Recent reports suggest that another form of vitamin A, retinyl palmitate, is potentially carcinogenic when used with sun protection. I am skeptical of this claim. In my opinion, the increased risk of cancer develops from the use of sunscreens and not from retinly palmitate. That being said, retinols have a 2 percent penetration rate. Unless this problem is overcome with a delivery mechanism like liposomes, retinols can be sun-sensitizing when they get lodged in the epidermis.

B VITAMINS

The B vitamins include several different vitamins. While all of them are beneficial, I believe vitamin B3 (niacinamide) is probably the most crucial to the skin because it increases the skin's own natural nutrition. In other words, it is able to increase the delivery of more nutrients to the dermis by increasing circulation. Again, this is more easily achieved if niacinamide is assisted by liposome delivery. Other B vitamins like panothenic acid, pyridoxine, and biotin are also beneficial to the skin.

VITAMIN C

I've talked extensively about vitamin C, but to recap: Vitamin C needs to be used in moderation, because, when it exists in excess in the epidermis, it can trigger inflammation and sun damage in the skin. Liposomal delivery is quite helpful, but equally as important is the use of non-oxidized vitamin C. This is only attainable if the vitamin C is mixed into a product in dry powder form. It is also important to use only L-ascorbic acid because that is the form that the skin responds to. In scientific terms, we should use what is called the "chirally correct" form of vitamin C.

VITAMIN D

Our skin produces vitamin D in response to ultraviolet exposure. It is an essential vitamin not only for the skin, but throughout the body. Unfortunately, a large portion of the population is deficient. That's why I recommend that people get 15 minutes a day of sunshine if possible. For even more benefit, vitamin D can be added via topical skincare products and internal supplementation.

VITAMIN E

Vitamin E is also very beneficial to the skin as it typically resides in the cell walls, helping to protect against cellular damage. It also rejuvenates vitamin C, amongst other activities. Vitamin E is another nutrient that you want to supplement orally.

MINERALS

The skin certainly can benefit from having minerals delivered to it, but the problem is that they can be strong irritants in the epidermis when used in high concentrations. As in the case of vitamins, topical minerals have a difficult time reaching the dermis. Yet products that employ liposomal delivery have much greater success.

ANTIOXIDANTS

Antioxidants are free-radical fighters, and therefore are key in our defense against numerous diseases. However, most antioxidants don't have very good penetration and many of them don't smell very good, so antioxidants typically aren't an effective addition to skincare products. Still, they are helpful and they do have some penetration ability, which is why I recommend a variety of antioxidants. The ones the skin uses most readily are superoxide dismutase, catalase, l-glutathione, coenzyme Q10, and R-lipoic acid. Liposome delivery increases the likelihood of dermal activity with these antioxidants.

AMINO ACIDS

Amino acids make up the building blocks of the nucleic acid in our DNA, in addition to collagen, antioxidants, peptides, and just about everything else in the skin. And body. That might lead you to believe that we have a plentiful supply, but because of vasoconstriction—oftentimes from stress, coffee, smoking, and aging—our circulation gets in the way of efficient amino acid delivery. Therefore, any strategy that increases circulation is going to increase the amount of amino acids. In addition, it's a good idea to enhance the delivery of amino acids by applying them to the skin. Research has shown that applying amino acids topically can improve the skin in several ways. The amino acids I recommend are proline, lysine, glycine, histidine, methionine, cysteine, glutamate, valine, leucine, and tryptophan. The skin uses these quite effectively in the capacity most needed. By using this approach, we are not mandating directional use for the amino acids through some kind of a peptide, but rather giving the skin the individual nutrients it needs to operate optimally.

LIPIDS

Lipids are another component that should be applied to the skin. As we have already discussed, many people believe, intuitively, that ceramides are the best lipid for the skin. However, it turns out that, because ceramides are chemical messengers in the epidermis, they cannot be used effectively without interrupting normal epidermal barrier turnover. Alternatives include linoleic acid, linolenic acid, cholesterol, and phosphatidylcholine. I prefer the use of phosphatidylcholine because it has dual functionality as both a liposome-delivery system as well as a lipid-replacement system. Applying lipids to the skin will definitely improve barrier function and hydration. It also normalizes oil production, along with preventing UVB damage. However, oils like olive oil have the propensity to oxidize and therefore have negative effects on the skin. I recommend using lipid components rather than straight oil in most cases.

To Sum It Up

To keep your skin healthy, you must eat nutritious foods and keep your digestive system functioning properly. However, many of us eat processed foods filled with toxic chemicals that do not nourish our bodies. Instead, these foods cause irritation and inflammation in the digestive tract, impeding its vital function. If you commit to changing your eating habits, you can ease digestive issues, clear up skin problems, and reduce the risk of many diseases such as diabetes and cancer.

Thanks to our fast-paced culture, Americans eat quickly and don't chew their food thoroughly. As a result, the enzymes in our mouth don't break down foods sufficiently and our stomach is not given adequate time to respond with the acids or enzymes needed to digest the foods properly. If you slow down and chew your food thoroughly, your digestion will improve. I also believe that eating different types of foods (i.e., carbohydrates and protein) together at one sitting disrupts digestion and leads to chronic conditions like constipation, diarrhea, acid reflux, and various skin conditions.

We all know junk food is unhealthy—so why can't we stop eating it? The simple answer is that we have become addicted to toxic and inflammatory foods because of the momentary high they give us. But we must change this bad habit. Our bodies function better when we don't consume inflammation-causing, nutrient-poor processed foods like bleached flour, refined sugars, preservatives, alcohol, and hydrogenated fats. For optimal digestion and nutrient absorption, you should also begin eating easily digestible foods; locally grown foods that are not filled with preservatives; organic fruits, vegetables, dairy, and meat; whole grains; good fats; and mineral supplements. I also recommend that you get certain vitamins, minerals, antioxidants, and other nutrients through topical formulations that will benefit the skin.

Topical nutrition does have its challenges, because the barrier is an effective deterrent and antioxidants, vitamins, and minerals get stuck and cause inflammation that reduces the net benefit of the active ingredients. In addition, these metallic or sulfur-based ingredients can affect a product's "cosmetic elegance and scent." One thing has become clear to me with regard to topical nutrition, and that is the necessity of using all the key components simultaneously. In other words, repairing skin is like baking a cake: If you don't have all the ingredients, the end result is flawed. In the case of skincare, any one of the missing ingredients can result in much less activity overall. For example, when L-ascorbic acid is missing, many activities are shut down; when zinc is in short supply, there is a dramatic decline in the health of the skin. When everything works in concert, as is the case in the skin, it is very important to make sure it has what it needs to operate optimally.

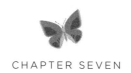

CHAPTER SEVEN

Sun and
Sun Protection

WHEN WE TALK ABOUT skin health, perhaps no subject receives more attention than the sun—and with good reason. Excess sun exposure is linked with wrinkles, leathery skin, age spots, and even skin cancer. So when dermatologists tell us to avoid the sun and slather on chemical sunscreens, we are inclined to follow their advice without question.

In recent years, though, plenty of research has come out that calls into question the wisdom of the medical consensus on sun safety and skin health. For instance, sun avoidance can cause insufficient vitamin D levels in the blood (the body converts the UV rays from the sun to vitamin D). This has been linked to numerous diseases, including osteoporosis and cancer. What's more, the sunscreens we've been religiously applying aren't simply ineffective, they are actually causing harm. One study found that people using sunscreen have significantly more inflammation in the skin than those not using it. Another shows that non-melanoma skin cancer rates have increased significantly over the past 20 years. As mounting evidence shows the dangers of chemical sunscreens, one thing is clear—it's time for a new, sensible approach to sun safety.

The sunscreens we've been religiously applying aren't simply ineffective, they are actually causing harm.

The Basics of Sunlight

The sun produces different types of light, but the ones of most concern are ultraviolet A (UVA) and ultraviolet B (UVB) rays. With new research, our understanding of UVA and UVB rays and how they affect the skin has changed. Experts once told us that only UVB damaged skin, but now we understand that UVA plays a role in premature skin aging and malignant melanoma.

Both UVA and UVB have short wavelengths, making them invisible to the naked eye. Approximately 95 percent of the radiation that reaches the earth from the sun is in the form of UVA rays. UVA penetrates the skin more deeply than UVB. It also can reach us through clouds and glass.

UVA rays are thought of as "tanning rays," and are the primary type of light used in tanning booths. Although some people think that a tan looks "healthy," it is actually the skin's self-protective reaction to UV light. When UV rays enter the skin, they damage the cells' DNA. This triggers the production of melanin over the two days that follow in an attempt to prevent further damage.

Over time, excess exposure to UVA rays causes wrinkling and other age-related skin decline. Research also shows that UVA rays can contribute to or even cause skin cancer. People who use tanning beds are far more likely to develop skin cancer, including malignant melanoma—the most deadly form of the disease.

UVB rays are thought of as the "burning rays." They reach us in the highest concentration between the hours of 10 a.m. and 4 p.m., and they are most intense from the months of April to October. People at high altitudes experience more exposure to UVB rays than people at lower elevations. With a shorter wavelength than UVA, UVB radiation penetrates only the outermost parts of the skin. However, it is still very damaging, which is why it is the primary culprit in most skin cancers.

How the Skin Responds to UV Radiation

The skin is very well designed. It knows that a certain amount of sun is both expected and needed on a daily basis. It also knows that with the benefits of sun come inevitable damage and inflammation. For this reason, the skin maintains an adequate supply of antioxidants, mineral cofactors, and other nutrients to repair any damage that may occur for a finite period of time.

The darker your complexion, the more the melanin in your skin minimizes inflammation. This explains why a 60-year-old African-American has fewer wrinkles than his Caucasian counterpart. When UVA/UVB rays penetrate past our protective pigment, they immediately begin creating inflammation. Fortunately, our skin responds quickly to begin the process of repairing damage to the DNA and other cellular components. That is why most of us can spend 10 to 15 minutes in the sun without developing a sunburn.

Clearly both UVA and UVB radiation incite short- and long-term damage to the skin. Effects range from the benign and cosmetic (like wrinkles and age spots), to serious and health-threatening effects like cancer. The exact mechanisms of these changes aren't entirely known, but research points to several ways in which UV radiation damages skin:

- **BREAKDOWN OF COLLAGEN AND ELASTIN.** Our skin is constantly making new collagen and elastin in the dermis. Collagen is the protein that gives skin its strength, and elastin gives it its elasticity. UV light causes damage to both. This results in the release of metalloproteinases (MMPs)—enzymes designed to break down the damaged collagen so the body can replace them with healthy collagen. While MMPs have been associated with aging, it's inaccurate to link them to dermal thinning. There is no scientific evidence to indicate that MMPs break down healthy skin. The thinning skin associated with age occurs when the skin sustains more damage than the body can repair. As we get older, we have less ability to create collagen and elastin at the levels needed to replace the damaged skin. This damaged collagen and elastin accumulate, leaving the dermis as a depository of waste that can also interfere with normal repair.

- **FREE-RADICAL DAMAGE.** We hear about the effects of free radicals on our bodies all the time. They're the reason we're encouraged to eat antioxidant-rich foods like berries and leafy greens. What we don't often hear about is that free-radical damage is among the main causes of skin damage—and that excess sun exposure can causes free radicals to form in the skin. As you may remember, free radicals are unstable oxygen molecules. Instead of having two electrons, these molecules have only one—which leaves them looking for extra electrons wherever they can find them. When free radicals exist in the body, they scavenge extra electrons from other cells, thus turning those cells into free radicals in search of a second electron. As this process repeats, it damages our cells and alters our DNA. In the skin, free-radical damage causes wrinkles and cancer. The skin knows it needs oxygen for survival, so it has built-in protective mechanisms to neutralize free radicals once they are created. These antioxidants can do their job until they are depleted, and then serious damage occurs.

- **DAMAGE TO THE DERMAL-EPIDERMAL JUNCTION.** The problem of free-radical damage is made worse by the fact that UV radiation damages the junction between the dermal and epidermal layers of the skin. All the antioxidants and nutrients the epidermis needs come from the dermis. When this connection is damaged, antioxidant delivery is hindered. That prevents the skin from being able to ward off free radicals effectively.

- **IMMUNE SYSTEM SUPPRESSION.** The skin is the body's first immune defender. UV radiation suppresses the skin's immune cells, making them less able to fight invaders and cells that are becoming cancerous. This is why any ingredient, including those in chemical sunscreens, should not create inflammation in already challenged skin.

These changes at the cellular level have drastic results—some of which can be seen in the mirror. The most immediate results of sun exposure are sunburns and tans, but those heal or fade. Over time, however, the damage caused to the skin can have other visible results.

- **DISCOLORATION.** UV rays activate melanocytes, which are the skin's pigment-producing cells. Repeated UV exposure damages the melanocytes' DNA, causing them to produce too much pigment (also called melanin). It can also cause the melanocytes to clump together, making that area of the skin darker. Another cause of discoloration occurs around the dermal-epidermal junction, where research has shown that debris builds up below the melanocyte. This likely results in a reduction of antioxidant delivery. All three causes lead to more pigment and resultant discoloration, more commonly known as freckles and age spots. On the flip side, UV exposure can also cause melanocytes to stop producing melanin, which results in light or white spots on the skin.
- **TEXTURE CHANGES.** In an almost adaptive response, repeated UV exposure can cause a thickening of the skin. This occurs as a result of injury to keratinocytes—skin cells that produce keratin. Although the skin is very good at repairing the epidermal cells, over time and repeated damage, it may develop problems with its protective barrier and become tough or leathery.
- **WRINKLES.** As previously discussed, the damage to collagen and elastin over time results in a progressive loss of structural support that leads to thinning of the dermis, wrinkles, and sagging skin.

While all of these concerns are benign, they can be upsetting from a cosmetic perspective. However, other skin concerns can be much more serious.

Sun Exposure and Skin Cancer

As we've established, excessive UV radiation damages the skin's cellular DNA. The genetic mutations that result can eventually lead to skin cancer.

Skin cancer is most common among fair-skinned people, who produce less melanin—the body's natural defense against sun damage.

There are three main types of skin cancer: basal cell carcinoma, squamous cell carcinoma, and malignant melanoma. Let's learn about each one.

- **Basal cell carcinoma** is the most common skin cancer, accounting for 75 percent of all skin cancers. It rarely metastasizes to other organs because it grows slowly. Basal cell carcinoma is linked to intermittent, intense sun exposure, especially during childhood and adolescence.

- **Squamous cell carcinoma** accounts for approximately 20 percent of all skin cancers, making it the second most common type of skin cancer. It is more likely than basal cell carcinoma to spread to other organs, but that's still rare. Squamous cell carcinoma is associated with chronic UVB exposure, rather than intermittent.

- **Melanoma** is the most dangerous of all skin cancers because it is much more likely to metastasize. Like basal cell carcinoma, melanoma is linked to intermittent and intense exposure, particularly before the age of 20. While melanoma can be deadly—it causes more than 8,000 deaths in the United States each year—it is highly curable if caught early.

Research shows that incidences of all three types of skin cancer have increased dramatically in the last 20 years.

Sun Protection

Given all we know about the damage that UV radiation causes to the skin, it's no wonder we're constantly looking for ways to protect ourselves from the sun. Dermatologists, on the whole, are strong advocates of sun avoidance and the copious use of sunscreens. It seems like a logical recommendation, since sunscreens do reduce sunburns and some sun-related skin conditions like actinic keratosis. But do they also prevent sun damage and skin cancer?

Unfortunately, research on the efficacy of sunscreens is less than compelling. Consider this fact: Since the early 1970s, when sunscreens started gaining in popularity, new cases of malignant melanoma have increased approximately 150 percent. In addition, studies have found that people who use more sunscreen have even higher rates of malignant melanoma. Recent research suggests that basal cell and squamous call carcinomas are also rising significantly.

A CLOSER LOOK AT SUNSCREENS

Sunscreens prevent sunburn by absorbing UV light. This reduces UV damage initially and prevents sunburn. Sunscreens have also been associated with reducing the incidence of actinic keratosis (pre-cancerous lesions). But sunscreen isn't benign. Some sunscreen chemicals—particularly avobenzone—can create free radicals when they are exposed to UV light. In addition, sunscreens can cause estrogenic side effects in the body, as well as inflammatory changes in the skin that could actually increase skin cancer occurrences and aging. No study is more telling of the quandary we face in deciding how to protect ourselves than the one in which researchers found increased inflammation in the skin of people using sunscreens than in those not wearing it. Evidence of estrogenic effects and the related toxicity is accumulating, though the actual mechanism is still not well understood. With all of the questions surrounding sunscreens, the trend is still for more, with SPF 100 now on retail shelves in America.

Sunscreens Versus Sunblocks

When it comes to topical sun protection products, you have two choices: sunscreen or sunblock. Sunscreens are chemical agents that actually absorb the sun's rays; sunblocks are minerals that reflect the rays. There are only two sunblocks currently being used: titanium dioxide and zinc oxide. Both of these naturally-occurring minerals provide good, broad-spectrum coverage of both UVA and UVB rays. Because sunscreens are designed to absorb the sun's rays, they are much more likely to break down into damaging byproducts than sunblocks. However, zinc and titanium also can become free radicals in the skin. (Remember that free radicals are unstable oxygen molecules that tear down DNA, cell walls, and much more.) Since zinc oxide has only one oxygen molecule, it will create half as much damage as titanium dioxide with its two oxygen molecules if and when it is broken down. Both of these molecules have less of a tendency to become free radicals in the skin because of their reduced absorption. The smaller (more "nano-sized") molecules look better on the skin but obviously penetrate better as well so there is a tradeoff.

I should clarify that the amount of inflammation form zinc and titanium is much lower than what is created by the breakdown of sunscreens.

some sunblocks, the minerals are coated with silica, which is an element that softens the skin and strengthens its connective tissue. But, when it coats zinc oxide or titanium dioxide, it serves another purpose: to prevent the minerals from becoming free radicals in the skin. For this reason, I am a fan of silica-coated zinc as the safest broad-spectrum protection currently on the market.

Not all sunblock comes in a tube, of course. Another common form of zinc oxide and titanium dioxide comes in the form of mineral makeup. This is often in a loose powder form, however, and when inhaled, titanium dioxide can contribute to a serious disease caused lung fibrosis. Zinc does not carry the same risks, so I prefer zinc-only mineral makeup.

Why Worry About Chemical Sunscreens?

As you might have figured out, I am not a fan of chemical sunscreens. I worry that they were rushed to market without sufficient studies being done on their efficacy and safety. Plus, many of the ingredients in chemical sunscreens have been proven to have detrimental effects on the skin and the body. Here are just a few of the chemicals of concern:

- **BENZOPHENONE** and its variants, dixoybenzone and oxybenzone, are common sunscreen ingredients. Oxybenzone was found to be safe in the 1970s, when sunscreens first started gaining in popularity. However, new research suggests that it might not be. Studies have linked it to allergies, hormone disruption, and cell damage. In addition, baby girls whose mothers are exposed to oxybenzone during pregnancy are at higher risk of being born at a low birth weight.

- **PABA (OR PARA-AMINOBENZOIC ACID) AND PABA ESTERS** (including ethyl dihydroxy propyl PAB, glyceryl PABA, padimate-O or octyl dimethyl PABA) have historically been very popular sunscreen ingredients, but as evidence against them grows—PABA is linked with allergic dermatitis, increased sensitivity to light (yes, you read that right), and cancer—many manufacturers are avoiding them. You'll still see padimate-O in a lot of sunscreens; it's supposedly less risky than PABA, but even that has been linked with free-radical formation.

~

Unfortunately, by protecting our skin
from sunburn with these chemical sunscreens,
we're causing other damage to DNA and likely
increasing our risk of skin cancer.

~

- CINNAMATES (CINOXATE, ETHYLHEXYL P-METHOXYCINNAMATE, OCTOCRYLENE, OCTYL METHOXYCINNAMATE) are the chemicals that are most frequently used in the United States to absorb UVB rays. Unfortunately, some cinnamates are known to cause allergic reactions in the skin when exposed to the sun on top of their free-radical production. Lab studies have also shown that cinnamates have estrogenic effects and can disrupt thyroid hormone and brain signaling.
- SALICYLATES (ETHYLHEXYL SALICYLATE, HOMOSALATE, OCTYL SALICYLATE) absorb UVB rays, but they are suspected of being hormone disruptors and forming toxic substances in the body.
- MENTHYL ANTHRANILATE is used as a UVA protector in some sunscreens. Europe and Japan both prohibit its use. Research suggests that it produces damaging free radicals when exposed to sunlight.
- AVOBENZONE (BUTYL-METHYOXYDIBENZOYLMETHANE; PARSOL 1789) is a popular sunscreen ingredient, used for absorbing UVA rays. It is the only chemical sunscreen ingredient allowed by the European community, but even it has limited protective abilities because it breaks down into unknown chemicals quickly.

As you can see, chemical sunscreens introduce a lot of risks in the name of protecting us from sun damage. Still, people are drawn to them. No wonder—sunburns are painful and they can cause serious, long-term damage to the skin. Unfortunately, by protecting our skin from sunburn with these chemical sunscreens, we are causing other damage to our DNA and likely increasing our risk of skin cancer.

That's right: The very lotion that you use on yourself and your family to prevent skin cancer is probably a contributor to the global epidemic of rising skin cancer rates. Skin cancer thrives on two things: DNA damage and weakened immune function. Evidence suggests these chemical sunscreens result in further damage to DNA, as well as inflammation—and excess inflammation weakens immune activity. Add to that the studies suggesting that both basal cell carcinoma and malignant melanoma rates are higher in individuals who routinely use chemical sunscreens, and we've cast some serious doubt on the risk-benefit argument in favor of these products.

In addition to cancer risk, many of the ingredients listed above have estrogenic effects in the body. What does estrogenic mean? Simply put, it means that the byproducts of these chemicals resemble part of an estrogen molecule. This means they can activate estrogen receptors in various parts of the body. For men, estrogen-mimickers can cause lower sperm counts, sexual identity confusion (male feminization), breast enlargement, and testicular cancer. Male fetuses and infants exposed to estrogenic chemicals are at risk for reduced penis size, undescended testicles, hypospadias, reduced libido, and feminized male behavior. In women, estrogenic chemicals can lead to endometriosis, migraines, reduced libido, severe PMS, altered menstrual cycles, reduced fertility, fibroids, fibrocystic breast disease, and uterine and breast cancer. It's worth noting that most of the research into the effects of estrogenic compounds on the body was conducted on other chemicals. However, ample research shows these sunscreen byproducts to be estrogenic and easily absorbed into our body—and given how much of it we apply to our skin every year, there's plenty of reason to be concerned. The epidemiological studies tracking the incidence of all of these conditions are quite alarming. The most rapid rise in cancer rates has occurred in hormone-related organs like ovaries, breast, prostate, and testes. Rates of undescended testes and hypospadias (congenital urinary tract defect) have doubled, and sperm counts have been cut almost in half.

Of course, sunscreens can't shoulder the blame for all of these changes. During the same time period, our world has been inundated with estrogenic pesticides and various other environmental toxins.

~

Ample research shows these sunscreen byproducts
to be estrogenic and easily absorbed into our body—
and given how much of it we apply to
our skin every year, there's plenty of reason
to be concerned.

~

However, the chemicals in sunscreens can stay in our bodies for years and have the potential to do serious damage. Studies even show notable levels of chemical sunscreens in breast milk as well, which is why I now advise expecting women to avoid chemical sunscreens while pregnant and/or breastfeeding.

The Sun Protection Factor

All sunscreens are labeled with their SPF, or Sun Protection Factor. This measures the amount of UVB radiation needed to cause sunburn with the sunscreen on, compared to the amount required to burn without it. You might think that, if you want to prevent sun damage, a higher SPF value would offer more protection. Unfortunately, SPF does not take into account the damage done by UVA rays, and it fails to account for the damage done by sunscreens after sun exposure. The higher the SPF, the higher the levels of estrogenic and inflammatory ingredients, though the amount of additional protection does not increase dramatically. For example, SPF 15 absorbs 93 percent of UVB rays, whereas SPF 30 absorbs 97 percent, and SPF 50 absorbs 98 percent. I recommend sticking with SPF 15 protection. This allows the average person the ability to stay in the sun three-plus hours without getting burned (which is enough for most). It also minimizes the exposure to toxic chemicals that will be absorbed into the body.

The other deceptive aspect of SPF is its lack of UVA protection. Without the burning rays providing us with a warning to get out of the sun, we tend to stay outdoors longer. Many people also mistakenly associate the lack of sunburn with complete protection.

~

The higher the SPF, the higher the levels
of estrogenic and inflammatory ingredients,
but the amount of additional protection does not
increase dramatically.

~

Broad-spectrum sunblocks, which protect against both UVA and UVB rays, in theory offer protection against the full spectrum of UV light. Titanium and zinc are effective in that regard, but they need constant reapplication. This makes them a challenge if you are swimming or perspiring. For this reason, most people select a combination product that has both a sunscreen for UVB protection and a UVA blocker. Unfortunately, UVA blockers wash off easily, leaving the skin exposed again. Unfortunately, these sunscreen users often do not realize they are only being protected from UVB after their initial dip in the pool.

The Future of Sun Protection

It's clear that something needs to change in the world of sun protection. One development I'm excited about is a new peptide that shows tremendous promise in protecting skin from the sun's harmful rays. This peptide, Skin Repair Growth Factor 7 (SRGF-7), uses "zinc finger" technology, which allows it to work at the cellular level to provide protection from sun exposure and sun damage. This peptide could completely change the sunscreen landscape because it is composed of amino acids, small amounts of zinc, and vitamin C—and yet it provides the equivalent of SPF 14 protection without any of the harmful side effects found in other sunscreens. Instead of absorbing UV light like other chemical sunscreens, SRGF-7 protects the skin and, more specifically, cellular DNA, by reducing cellular inflammation. As an added benefit, it can help heal sunburns after they've already occurred. Early indications show that this very same zinc finger technology may also have beneficial effects on actinic keratosis and skin cancer.

Nano-Sized Particles—Good or Bad?

Throughout the skincare universe, particles keep getting smaller and smaller. The main reason for this is to increase penetration and absorption. However, these tiny particles (called nanoparticles) are so small that they can travel, almost unmitigated, throughout the body. Nano-sized zinc and titanium are commonly found in sunblocks, and they've been shown to provide a better level of sun protection than larger-sized versions of the same molecules. Because zinc is prevalent in our cells and tissues, I'm not concerned about the absorption of nano-sized zinc into our bloodstream. However, I think we are asking for trouble when using nano-sized titanium. Although we all get trace amounts of this mineral in our diets, higher levels can be toxic. I recommend caution when using sunblocks with nano-sized titanium.

Another intriguing area of research is Harmonized Water. Harmonized Water is water that has been imbued with specific radio frequencies designed to serve different purposes. One of those frequencies allows the water to neutralize the effects of UV light. When you ingest the water, the energetic frequency spreads to the skin within an hour and lasts for about three hours. It then provides the equivalent of SPF 15 protection for three-plus hours. While for some this may simply be additional sun protection to support topical creams, darker skin types may find this to be all they need. There are also some antioxidant products on the market that when ingested can offer moderate sun protection, as well.

Toward a Sensible Sun-Protection Plan

In order to spend time in the sun safely, I recommend this sensible sun-safe plan.

- **APPLY ZINC SEVERAL TIMES A DAY** as needed when you're in the sun. As I've said, I believe that sunblocks are safer than the chemical sunscreens on the market, and zinc oxide is safer than titanium diox-ide. However, zinc cannot be made water-resistant or waterproof, so we need to apply it very frequently when we're in the water or when we're perspiring.

- **WEAR SUN-PROTECTIVE CLOTHING.** Sun shirts are a wonderful invention. They can provide SPF 10–15 protection and can get wet and be worn all day. Best of all, they provide even protection, with no gaps or missed spots. Unfortunately, they don't help protect the face, hands, and legs.
- **USE SUNSCREENS AS LITTLE AS POSSIBLE.** Even with sun shirts, the face and (sometimes) legs often need to have protection that survives the many dunks in the pool or a day of spring skiing. If water-resistance is the key, only sunscreens have staying power.
- **TRY HARMONIZED WATER.** This water carries a specific energetic frequency that can mitigate the sun's damaging effects on the body. It bypasses the issue of water-resistance and has proven to be remark-ably effective in most people.
- **LOOK FOR SRGF-7**. Because SRGF-7 shows promise in calming cellular inflammation and protecting DNA—and because it does not break down into free radical–forming molecules or estrogenic com-pounds when exposed to the sun—this is one of the most exciting developments in sun protection.

Don't forget, sun exposure is good! With all the talk about wrin-kles, DNA damage, and skin cancer, it's easy to forget that our bodies actually need the sun—it's not the enemy we sometimes perceive it to be. It's important that we find a way to reap the sun's benefits while minimizing its risks. In order to maintain optimal vitamin D levels in the body, we need to spend at least 15 minutes a day in the sun—up to three more if you are dark-skinned. Research has shown that daily sunshine reduces your incidence of breast cancer, colon cancer, and osteoporosis; increases serotonin levels; improves immunity; lowers blood pressure and cholesterol; improves sex drive; and regulates sleep patterns. So be sure to get out and enjoy the sunshine safely—it does a body good.

To Sum It Up

For decades, dermatologists have warned us to either avoid the sun or slather on chemical sunscreens any time its rays hit our bare skin. But recent research questions this approach because blocking sun exposure leads to a lack of vitamin D. This, in turn, increases the risk of many serious diseases. Also, the sunscreens we apply every day may not be as effective as we thought at protecting us from harmful rays. Even more concerning, some sunscreens contain toxic chemicals linked to cancer, hormone disruption, allergies, and dermatitis. And it's important to understand that, because these chemicals damage DNA, create inflammation, and weaken your immune system, the very thing you are applying to stave off skin cancer could be increasing your risk of the disease.

I believe it's time to rethink our approach to sun protection. I recommend ditching chemical sunscreens for silica-coated zinc oxide sunblock—the safest broad-spectrum protection currently available. But because it's not water-resistant, you must remember to apply it several times a day when you're enjoying the water or perspiring. Titanium dioxide is another naturally occurring mineral that provides good, broad-spectrum coverage of both UVA and UVB rays, but it creates a little more free-radical damage in your skin than zinc oxide. I also recommend a new peptide, Skin Repair Growth Factor 7 (SRGF-7), which uses "zinc finger" technology and works at the cellular level to protect your skin from sun damage. And lastly, as an adjunct to everything else, Harmonized Water is an exciting new development.

Part 4

~

Solutions for Problem Skin

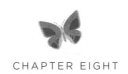

CHAPTER EIGHT

Turning Back
the Clock

~

A critical long-term strategy for aging must be to
minimize inflammation wherever possible.

~

ONE THING READERS AND practitioners alike must understand is
that the skin is specifically designed to handle damage, even excessive
damage, quite well. Our goal should be to assist and support the skin
in carrying out its function. A critical long-term strategy for aging
must be to minimize inflammation wherever possible. This will allow
the skin to manage the inflammation that is unavoidable throughout
our lifetimes.

African-American skin presents us with a relevant case in point on
the topic of inflammation and aging. As I discussed earlier, African-
American skin naturally maintains an SPF value of approximately 13.4.
It is worth observing that 13.4 SPF does not block all of the UV rays
from the sun, but it does protect against roughly 90 percent of them.
While African-American skin has a higher tolerance for sun exposure, to
suggest that African-American skin is immune to the effects of the sun is
inappropriate. Analysis of African-Americans reveals that their skin does
in fact suffer a fair amount of DNA damage from sun exposure.

Given what we know about melanin and pigmentation, you might look at African-American skin and assume that it never gets inflamed. In truth, *everybody's* skin takes a tremendous beating from excessive sun, and African-Americans enjoy no exception from this rule. What is of interest, however, is that African-American skin can take a fairly aggressive beating yet still exhibit considerably less sun damage compared with Caucasian skin types. As I discuss elsewhere in the book, African-Americans generally can make it to age 60 before developing facial wrinkles. They are 13 times less likely to develop malignant melanoma and 50 times less likely to get basal cell and squamous cell carcinomas. So despite the effects of harsh sun exposure, we can conclude that our skin can handle a lot of inflammation before it begins to lose collagen and elastin. It is only the extreme excesses from which it does not recover fully. For lighter skin types, unfortunately, those excesses come much more frequently, which results in early aging effects.

In addition to understanding that the skin is designed to handle inflammation (so long as we don't add fuel to the fire through our interventions and treatment methods), we must also remember that human beings are genetically designed to function out of doors. If our skin could not tolerate UV light, then of course we would find ourselves in a very difficult situation. But we *can* tolerate moderate amounts of UV radiation and, as a point of fact, some sun exposure every day is critical to our overall health and to our skin's health. With this in mind, let's not approach aging with a deeply formed fear of the sun's effects on our skin. Instead, let's examine the ways in which we may enjoy our time outside, both by allowing for appropriate amounts of UV exposure and by protecting against excessive amounts of the same exposure.

~

The epidermis is actually designed to
reflect 80 percent of the sunlight that hits it.
That's pretty remarkable when
you consider the intensity of the sun.

~

The Skin's Defense Mechanisms

We know that human skin has several built-in defense mechanisms to deal with the inflammation it is bound to absorb over time. The first mechanism is the barrier itself. The skin's epidermal barrier takes the brunt of the damage. The dermis also bears the weight of inflammation over time, but to a lesser degree.

The epidermis is actually designed to reflect 80 percent of the sunlight that hits it. That's pretty remarkable when you consider the intensity of the sun. Of course, the remaining 20 percent of light that penetrates the epidermis must be dealt with. The skin, as we'll explore, is designed to deal with this exposure and the resulting inflammation.

Once sunlight has penetrated the epidermis, questions of melanin production become especially relevant. Each of us possesses a unique genetic code that determines the amount of melanin we produce. Interestingly, all of us have roughly the same quantity of melanocytes, or melanin-producing cells, per square inch of skin, regardless of whether we are black, brown, red, pink, yellow, orange, or blue. What changes from person to person, however, is how much melanin those cells are genetically capable of producing. As you have guessed by now, darker skin types, such as African-Americans and Latinos, produce more melanin than do Caucasians. Of course, the average brown-haired Caucasian produces more melanin than the average blonde or redhead, who produce more melanin than an albino.

Once we understand the geographical reasons for skin color and skin tone, then, on a spectrum of melanin production, we can begin to understand the inherent risks we face if our exposure levels fail to align with our natural melanin levels. If we were to graph the ideal sun-exposure-to-skin-type ratio, with minutes of exposure on the "Y" axis and skin type on the "X" axis, we could each identify the sweet spot, given our varying genetic predispositions for melanin production, for the amount of sunlight we may reasonably tolerate without causing undue damage. Genetically determined melanin content shifts based on the amount and intensity of sun exposure to which a region is exposed. For example, Northern European skin gets very little intense sunlight and so the body reduces melanin for two reasons: to allow more efficient manufacturing of vitamin D and because the skin does not need to waste its resources. Whereas, African skin requires more exposure for adequate vitamin D production, but the focus of the melanin increase is survivability in the intense, hot sun of that continent. When our skin is designed to be in one region of the world and we migrate to another, our inadequate, innate protection system fails us—and aging and disease become more prevalent. Such awareness is beneficial for us all, as the amount of melanin production helps to determine an individual's risk of skin cancer, the onset of wrinkles, and other signs of aging.

Just as melanin is one essential repair mechanism imbued in the skin, so, too, is the system that produces antioxidants to neutralize free radicals generated by the sun and other damage. Just as melanin levels vary from group to group and from individual to individual, so, too, do antioxidant production levels. Everyone's body produces varying levels of antioxidants, including l-glutathione, superoxide dismutase, and catalase, based on individual need. We all know someone with average melanin activity who still has strikingly smooth and youthful skin for her age but has been exposed to similar levels of UV as her contemporaries. This person, we can surmise, produces enviable antioxidant counts that help the skin to age well.

Immune function is another factor in aging, and the skin has its own immune function as a part of the body's systems. We all know people who never seem to get sick, people who can eat anything and not gain weight, or people who seem to heal from illness or injury faster than the rest of us. In the same vein, some of us have higher levels of immune function relative to the skin (and most likely overall, as systemic health is related throughout the body). These people are often healthy and most likely work to stay that way, but they also enjoy a genetic aptitude for repairing and maintaining the skin. As a result, such individuals will likely be perceived to age well, especially where the skin is concerned. As should be expected, if we live lifestyles that suppress our immune function, we can expect an impeded immune response in the skin.

Signs and Symptoms of Aging Skin

As we age, the skin goes through a continual transformation. When and to what extent we experience the signs and symptoms of aging varies from person to person, but we'll all experience one or more of the following changes as we get older.

WRINKLES

The first indicator of skin aging is the appearance of wrinkles. For fairer skin types, wrinkles develop some time around the age of 30. As we've discussed already, individuals with higher melanin productivity and those who produce greater levels of antioxidants naturally will make it far longer without experiencing wrinkles. The timing is dependent, of course, on their specific levels of melanin and antioxidants, as well as on the number of times excess UV exposure occurred in their lifetime.

While wrinkles appear to be a problem at the surface of the skin, they actually form as a result of lost elastic capacity and lost collagen density at the dermal level. Recall that the dermis thins at a rate of 1 percent per year after the age of 20. This thinning, which is inevitable, is something of a structural collapse of the collagen that previously maintained our skin's surface wrinkle-free. Without the structural integrity once provided by robust collagen supports, wrinkles will develop.

As collagen breaks down over time, the dermis actually becomes more fluid-like where it was once more solid in nature. We see this first in areas of facial expression: around the eyes, on the forehead, between the eyebrows, around the mouth, and perhaps farther out on the cheeks. These wrinkles appear first as we age because these are the areas of the dermis most frequently exposed to compression. Of course, we are expressive long before we reach our 30s, but as we age and collagen begins to break down, our once-resilient skin gives way to the passage of time.

The muscles in the face are actually quite strong. When they compress or contract, they push the more-fluid dermal tissue out of the way. When we're young, we have plenty of collagen and elastin, so compression is not an issue for the skin. The rigid nature of the collagen and the elastic nature of the elastin give our skin both the strength and the dynamic it needs to return to normal (smooth) after smiling or frowning. Later in life, as collagen density deteriorates, the once-immobile dermis becomes more malleable, and wrinkles appear.

As we get older and collagen density within the dermal matrix diminishes, we observe a much slower recovery of the gap that forms the wrinkle. What happens at this time is that, when we smile, we push the fluid matrix and essentially split it into two different sections. With repetitive expression, the gap has the tendency to stay in place even after our facial muscles have ceased to contract.

One option is to stop making the expressions—stop contracting the muscles, that is—that cause wrinkles. When the muscles no longer exert force on the compromised dermis, we actually see that the skin equilibrates, or balances out, and the net result is that a specific wrinkle can diminish pretty quickly. This is why Botox works. Botox stops the facial contraction and allow the dermal fluid matrix to balance and smooth out rather than split in two under pressure from facial muscles. This is also why devices like a microcurrent or anything that is repeatedly pushed along the skin can give an "instant facelift." They push the dermal matrix around until some of the gaps (previously created by facial expression) are filled. Unfortunately, both approaches provide only temporary results because the skin still lacks structural support to prevent a new gap from forming.

FACIAL CAPILLARIES

Another symptom of aging skin is revealed in the form of facial capillaries. Traditionally, visible facial capillaries are most common among adults over 60. Lately, though, we've begun to see more individuals develop visible facial capillaries at younger ages—in their 30s, 40s, and 50s. These can result from the thinning of the dermis or possibly DNA damage. Facial capillaries are not necessarily part of rosacea, although the latter is a growing occurrence in this country. The chief complaint of rosacea sufferers routinely focuses on the network of capillaries that becomes visible beneath the surface of the skin. Rosacea ignites the capillaries as a response to inflammation. The skin registers inflammation as a symptom of inflammation elsewhere, usually in the gut. In response, vasodilation occurs to allow greater circulation to rush nutrients to affected areas. These capillaries are actually engorged, to a point, as the skin contends with inflammation.

Rosacea-related facial capillaries and facial capillaries that emerge as a result of aging are not the same.

On their own, visible facial capillaries appear as we age because, if you'll recall, the dermis thins at a rate of 1 percent a year after the age of 20. To be specific, we lose what is called the papillary dermis as a result of our inability to adequately restore damaged collagen. In the case of most facial capillaries, the skin simply thins enough to reveal any capillaries that happen to be extremely close to the skin's surface. The fact that certain capillaries do reside near surface level is not unusual, nor is their appearance cause for alarm. After all, many of these capillaries are important feeders of the epidermis and the heavily damaged areas of the papillary dermis. As we lose density in the dermis, these blood vessels become more exposed. Of course, for many of us, any sign of aging skin is cause for alarm, at least cosmetically. To this end, it's easier to promote overall skin health throughout our lifetimes than it is to chase visible capillaries around the face with a laser in the hopes of "restoring" a youthful appearance.

There is another aspect to facial capillaries that has yet to be fully examined. The idea of capillaries expanding as a result of DNA damage. Every aspect of the skin has been created by the reading and implementation of our genetic code. This includes the formation of blood vessels, immune cells, and everything else. It is not a big surprise to think that UV-ravaged skin could have errors in the process of new blood cell formation ("angiogenesis"). What led me to this conclusion was the remarkable effects zinc fingers have on facial capillaries. They are so effective that, a few weeks into therapy, many people have seen a clearance of their "broken capillaries."

UNEVEN SKIN TONE

Uneven skin tone is the result of a combination of red, white, and brown spots. Generally, we see brown spots develop first in places where melanocytes have been damaged or have clustered together resulting in melanin-production spikes in that specific region. This condition is known as hyperpigmentation. Conversely, as we age, we may observe inconsistent whitening of the skin in various places as hypopigmentation occurs. Hypopigmentation reflects the discontinuation of melanin production to cells in a specific area. This is usually an end-stage event symbolizing the loss of melanocytes in that area. Since melanocytes have stem cell reserves, it takes a long history of UV damage (or an overly traumatic procedure) to develop hypopigmentation.

We may also see red spots emerge on the skin, especially at points that have taken more extreme abuse from the sun. These spots can become actinic keratosis (pre-cancerous red/flakey lesions) or simply remain areas of smoldering inflammation. There is also a combined event where smoldering inflammation leads to the formation of more melanin. In fact, I have found a unique type of "age spot" that is particularly resistant to treatment. I believe there may be an association with liver damage that shows as an inflamed and pigmented spot on the skin. So the old wives' description of a "liver spot" may be accurate in some cases. Regardless of the coloring of the skin, when such unevenness appears the change serves as a reminder and a caution to us that those parts of the skin have undergone significant damage over time. That's why it's so important to protect all of our skin as we age, and especially the troubled spots described here.

Incidents of hyperpigmentation have been linked to a buildup of scar tissue along the dermal-epidermal junction. In such cases, hyperpigmentation appears to be, in part, the result of an inability to deliver antioxidants because of interference from cellular debris beneath the discolored area. Remember that antioxidants have to be delivered from the dermal supply; and, if they cannot pass through a region because there is an abnormally dense cell population, then the melanocyte will have to compensate by making more melanin. The dense cellular debris is found at the junction between the dermis and epidermis, and forms as a result of the repeated damage. It is only found under melanocytes that are hyperactive.

What should be worrisome to all of us as we age is that age-related hyperpigmentation is a warning sign that an area of the skin is coming under repeated fire, and that the area may be in trouble. If the skin produces excess melanin, then we must recognize that significant damage is already underway. We must also realize that the dermis is presumably sending antioxidants and other nutrients to the epidermis, but the epidermis *isn't receiving the help*. At this point, it is appropriate to change our behavior in order to help the skin avoid further damage. Blocking the sun, either with clothing, sunblock, or shade, becomes a priority if we wish to mitigate skin damage and allow the body to begin to heal itself. Lasers and peels may successfully lighten the affected skin, but they won't resolve the damage. Liposomal treatments can restore cellular integrity at the damaged site, and this is beneficial in the treatment of aging-related hyperpigmentation. Even liposomal therapy, however, is no substitute for prudence and care.

Unlike hyperpigmentation, which may be mitigated by not-so-perfect remedies like laser treatments or chemical peels, hypopigmentation often results in lasting discoloration. In general, when we see areas of the skin that have lost their ability to produce normal pigment, then we can assume that permanent damage has been sustained.

Redness, which we've also mentioned in this section, usually indicates that the skin is attempting to heal from some damage or injury. In such cases, the redness resolves itself over a period of months. Cases of chronic, ongoing redness indicate deeper and more serious damage to the skin's DNA. Often accompanied by flakiness, these cases should not be taken lightly, as a simple sign of aging. Such damage reflects a level of actinic keratosis and may be a precursor of cancer.

ENLARGED PORES AND GROWTHS

Pores serve the skin by allowing sweat and sebum, a naturally produced oil, to exit the skin and carry away toxins and debris. As we age, pores may enlarge as a result of excessive oil production or thinning skin. In moving toxins out of the body through the skin, the pores will take a hit and exhibit inflammation. The toxins we eliminate are not totally benign, and as they irritate and inflame the skin they may result in atrophy immediately around the pore.

Over time, the atrophy surrounding the pore becomes even more pronounced because we lose our collagen infrastructure in the dermis. Imagine that the hair follicle is a tent pole and the skin a tent. Even though the extruding hair is soft, the follicle root is fairly rigid, enough so that it causes the skin to be held up slightly. Over time, sagging in the skin around the follicle will occur. Without the stability previously provided by the presence of robust collagen levels, the epidermis collapses beside the pore, enhancing the appearance of enlargement. This appearance can be further exacerbated by dirt that collects in pores from the surface or by overactive sebaceous glands.

Fortunately, enlarged pores can be treated by rebuilding the collagen and elastin matrix in the dermis. Through stimulating collagen and elastin and by decreasing sebum output, we can significantly reduce the appearance of enlarged pores.

Growths on the skin represent another sign of aging. Skin tags, hemangiomas, and some moles—benign tumors—often signal a compromised immune system. Don't panic when you read "compromised immune system." My goal is to educate, not to scare. The truth is that, as we age, immune function declines. In our earlier years, the skin is more adept at resolving viruses, fungi, irritation, and inflammation that can lead to growths. New moles should not convince you that you've developed an autoimmune disease. But recognize that the skin is telling you, with the appearance of these little reminders, that you're not as young as you used to be and you may need to take greater precautions and cover up more of your skin with more regularity.

A Word About Hormones

Hormone levels obviously change as you age. Also, recognize that hormones play critical roles in day-to-day skin condition and appearance. Testosterone levels—in both men and women—dictate oil production and in turn contribute to acne, but testosterone can also stimulate collagen and elastin. Estrogen levels—again in both men and women—impact collagen and elastin production, and directly relate to skin integrity. We should not fret over hormonal shifts and their effects on the skin, but it is always beneficial to keep in mind all the variables that factor into the health of our skin. Understanding the ebb and flow of hormone levels throughout our lives may help us to gain perspective on our daily skincare battles. Women can see dramatic changes in their skin in relatively short periods of time as they enter menopause. Topical

Do Skin Tags Mean I Have HPV?

Skin tags, or small tumors that form on the skin, have long been a source of consternation and wonder. Known scientifically as acrochorda, skin tags may be cosmetically undesirable and inconvenient when shaving, but they are benign and present no significant health concerns. Because of their location in areas such as the neck, armpits, groin, underside of the breast, and similar regions, friction is identified as a culprit in the formation of skin tags in at least one report. Higher rates of skin-tag formation among obese persons support the idea that friction plays a role in their occurrence.

Questions abound as to a possible connection between skin tags and the human papilloma virus, commonly known as HPV. A 2008 study by researchers in India corroborates an earlier study suggesting an HPV link to the appearance of skin tags. HPV occurs in high-risk and low-risk strains. Fortunately, another 2008 study reports zero detection of high-risk HPV in skin tags among a group of child participants. So while emerging evidence supports a link between skin tags and low-risk HPV, skin tags in and of themselves should not signal concern over the high-risk strain of HPV associated with sexually transmitted disease.

I think their existence still stems from a virus, regardless of the studies presented. It may be HPV or another virus. The fact that these show up in areas that have friction may simply mean that friction, by compromising skin health, makes it easier for the virus to have an impact. Regardless, zinc finger technology appears to correct the virus' impact on our skin's DNA, and other procedures can remove them quite easily.

estrogen and progesterone will help, but they come with potential side effects. Phytoestrogens in topical formulas can help, but not always. I have seen great results from stem cell growth media in menopausal skin, but it is too early to know if these contain growth factors that counteract losses in systemic estrogen/progesterone or if they promote general skin-health improvement.

~

To help your skin age gracefully, protect the barrier.
Don't exfoliate. If you do exfoliate, stop today.

~

Care for Seasoned Skin

While the skincare market is rife with products, treatments, and regimens designed to baby your skin (and lighten your pocketbook) as you age, the best thing you can do for an aging dermis is to support the skin in all its stages. To this end, there are certain principles we should heed throughout our lives that will pay dividends years down the road. By protecting the barrier, encouraging melanin production, and increasing skin nutrition, we will extend the health and preserve the appearance of our skin well into our golden years.

For the past 30 or so years, Americans have held dear to the notion that exfoliation, whether by peel, scrub, or acid, should be part of the *daily* skin routine. This misguided notion could not be farther from the truth. The skin exfoliates at a perfect rate—even as that rate changes over time—based on the amount of nutrition it needs and the amount of damage it sustains. In other words, the skin is an intelligent organ that adapts to its environment. The epidermis acts as a two-way filter, keeping dirt and debris out and keeping appropriate levels of nutrients in until such time as the body is ready to dispose of them. To force your skin to exfoliate on a daily or weekly basis is to strip the skin of its barrier against harsh environmental irritants and to damage the insulator that ensures the dermis gets maximum sustenance from the nourishment we offer. Nothing could be more misguided, from the vantage point of skin health, than such extreme exfoliation.

Instead, we should protect the barrier. The outermost layer of the epidermis, the stratum corneum, is, aside from melanin, one of the best tools we have to protect us from the sun. Lipids, which reside in the oils that the skin naturally produces, are our best protection against surface inflammation. To practice daily removal of the outer epidermis and the lipids on the skin's surface is to cause inflammation and deterioration.

Ironically, exfoliation has an effect opposite to the one intended by most skincare professionals today. Rather than rejuvenating, it ages the skin. And when we strip oils from the skin and cause inflammation, the skin responds by increasing oil production to restore the barrier. This can result in "shiny" or oily skin. It is my contention that the "oily T-zone" was created by over-exfoliation. To help your skin age gracefully, protect the barrier. Don't exfoliate. If you do exfoliate, keep it to no more than once a month and make sure it involves limited trauma.

Next, respect that melanin. No matter what our thoughts on brown spots or uneven coloration may be, melanin is our best natural defense against sun damage. The strong acids we use in the course of exfoliation cause deeper damage to the skin's DNA at the cellular level. This damage, which also affects the melanocyte, often results in the abnormal production of "age spots." Part of the damage comes from the reduction of protective melanin in the skin when forced exfoliation is used regularly. In turn, we become more susceptible to harm from the sun. Any time we attempt to lighten our pigmentation, we increase inflammation to the skin immediately. There is simply no way to reconcile what we know about inflammation and cellular degeneration with practices such as exfoliating and lightening. These routines, which are the gold standard of current professional skincare practices, are guaranteed to increase and accelerate the signs of aging because they fail to protect the barrier and respect the role of melanin in defending the skin.

By protecting the barrier and promoting melanin production, we can help our skin age as gracefully as possible. Of course, most of us will still experience superficial damage, and many of us will experience deeper damage. Almost without exception, any treatment we undertake for any skin complaint will be more effective if we can also calm inflammation at the source.

Increasing Nutrition: Vasodilation and Liposomal Niacinamide

All of the skin's defense mechanisms—epidermal integrity, melanin production, antioxidant production, and immune function—factor in to the daily survival of the skin. Each component is critical to skin health vn right, but there is an overarching item missing from this list: uality and quantity of nutrients delivered to the skin can make eveɪ y difference in how our skin will age. None of the above-mentioned characteristics can attain maximum potential if the skin does not receive the nutrition it needs.

To this end, one thing we can do to maximize nutrient delivery to the skin is to dilate the blood vessels in the skin and increase circulation to the dermis. As we age, however, fewer and fewer capillaries will be available each year to nourish the dermis. Capillary function, unfortunately, is also reduced as a natural side effect of aging. As a result, the capillaries we are fortunate enough to hold on to can't deliver enough nutrition to keep the skin looking young. Capillaries, of course, are made of collagen. As collagen is damaged by the sun, capillaries actually develop scar tissue that surrounds them and negatively impacts the distribution of nutrients from the affected blood vessels. When we properly understand the role capillaries play in skin nutrition, we can really see the value of increasing circulation to counteract the effects of aging.

Where aging interventions are concerned, introduction of vasodilators is one of the best steps we can take to maintain skin function and appearance. Of available vasodilators, liposomal niacinamide is the most promising application on the market. In addition to dilating the blood vessels, niacinamide has been shown to improve the barrier of the skin, normalize pigmentation, clear acne, and prevent sun damage. Niacinimide has also been shown to promote collagen and elastin production. Delivered via liposome, niacinamide has the added benefit of working directly at the cellular level in the deeper skin layers to restore and enhance skin cells without becoming trapped in the epidermis. So not only can niacinamide boost nutrition to the skin, but it will result in a host of positive side benefits as well, including barrier protection, improvement in hyperpigmentation and acne, increased collagen production, and more.

To Sum It Up

Aging is one of those skin conditions we'll all have to reckon with over time. Fortunately, the skin is remarkably well-designed to handle inflammation and repair injuries sustained throughout a lifetime. Naturally, whether we like to acknowledge it or not, skin health deteriorates and resilience declines. As a result, even the healthiest among us will notice wrinkles, uneven coloration, facial capillaries, enlarged pores, skin tags, and more.

Protecting the barrier and encouraging melanin production are essential to helping the skin age well. Improving nutrient delivery is also critical and, outside of a healthy diet and strong circulation, liposomal technology can assist skin cells to get the nourishment they need.

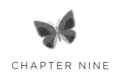

CHAPTER NINE

Skin Conditions, Common Approaches, and Preferred Treatments

What Goes In ...

In this chapter, we'll explore several of the more common skin conditions that drive consumers to seek treatment from dermatologists, aestheticians, and skincare products. I've mentioned these conditions throughout the book, but here we'll look more deeply into the how and why of such maladies like acne, rosacea, melasma, and more. With regard to each problem and diagnosis, we'll also look for internal clues about the body's general level of health, toxicity, and overall balance. Such considerations help us lessen or alleviate many skin complaints without resorting to topical treatments. Cleaning up the body from the inside out also clears away internal obstacles that may impede external results. The skin is, after all, an organ of detoxification; that is, when the body seeks to push toxins out of its various systems, many substances get released through the skin. In this way, what goes into the body is perfectly relevant to the conditions manifested on the skin.

Scientists are divided on the degree to which diet affects the skin's condition, but I do not waver in my assertion that processed foods that are high in sugar are culprits in a number of skin-related complaints. We are, in fact, largely addicted to foods that are arguably toxic to our bodies.

Some of us are addicted to caffeine, cigarettes, alcohol, or other drugs. Others are addicted to exercise for the release of beta-endorphins and adrenaline that result from a good workout. Similarly, many of us are addicted to food—aside from our need for nourishment—because of the "high" that results from surges of cortisol and beta-endorphins as we ingest common ingredients such as bleached flour, sugar, and alcohol.

Just as we've discussed the importance of avoiding inflammation topically—most commonly through over-exfoliation by one means or another—we must also avoid inflammatory foods, which cause inflammation throughout the body. Sugars and alcohol are among the most inflammatory substances we eat. Dairy is inflammatory inasmuch as it increases mucous production and acidity, though it does not inflame to the degree sugar and alcohol do.

The conditions that we'll discuss in this chapter, including acne, rosacea, melasma, hyperpigmentation, and aging, are all associated with inflammation of the skin. It makes sense, therefore, that minimizing inflammation internally will only help to reduce or alleviate the symptoms of systemic inflammation, as well as these skin conditions. Consuming foods filled with artificial ingredients, refined sugars, and preservatives, as well as drinking alcohol or sodas, creates inflammation and leaves our bodies unbalanced. By identifying and eliminating such substances from our diet, we can help the skin come into alignment with the systems of the body.

This chapter will also touch on how intestinal and bowel health contributes to healthy skin. Without going into gruesome detail, we must understand that any substances we ingest that are harmful to our system

~

In actuality, buying a bunch of organic kale
for a few dollars at your local farmers' market
will do more for your skin over time—
and do it more effectively—than a laser peel
or a tube of this season's miracle skin goo.

≈

Just as an individual would naturally ask for help moving a couch that is too big and heavy to carry alone, the skin sends out an urgent call for help to relieve the overgrowth in bacteria.

aren't just eliminated the next day. Although we have a pretty good filter system, experiencing toxicity from foods we eat is a common occurrence. Secondly, we don't want to create inflammatory byproducts from good foods, but we certainly do that when we hamper our digestive juices (see Chapter 6). Lastly, this abuse adds up over the years, leading to malabsorption, constipation, leaky gut, and other issues that increase inflammation in the body and often in the skin. Carefully choosing what we ingest helps to alleviate some of the heavy lifting our organs must do to sort nutrients from waste and process foodstuffs through our systems. The fewer toxins we put into our bodies, the fewer toxins we are ultimately tasked with getting out.

To this end, I cannot say enough about dietary fiber. It is so much easier to keep the bowel functioning smoothly than to encounter a backup, literally, which demands intervention. By the time waste accumulates and hardens on the bowel wall, the body has essentially stockpiled toxins that it was never designed to process through digestion and metabolization. An increased toxic load leads to immunosuppression, yeast overgrowth, and hormonal irregularities. These toxins leach into the bloodstream and poison us for years—yet we hardly acknowledge the burden this places on all the systems of the body. Instead, we too often look for solutions in designer packaging. In actuality, buying a bunch of organic kale for a few dollars at your local farmers' market will do more for your skin over time—and do it more effectively—than a laser peel or a tube of this season's miracle skin goo.

Our digestive tract is responsible for more than 60 percent of our immune function, so when its health declines, so does the rest of the body. While specific foods may or may not trigger skin events, your overall health is impacted by the (often compromised) environment of the digestive system. It should also not be surprising that changes happening along the digestive wall are mirrored by the skin in many cases.

So let's take a closer look at the skin conditions that plague many of us at different stages in our lives.

Acne

So many of us will deal with acne at some time in our lives. To understand how acne occurs, we must first appreciate that the human body is covered in hair. True, most of our hair is of the vellus variety, which means that the hairs are small, fine, and light in color. We largely don't see these hairs when we look at the skin from a distance. But the average person's skin is actually covered in some five million hairs, each of which sprouts from a hair follicle three to four millimeters beneath the surface of the skin. These hair follicles serve a tremendous function. In addition to facilitating hair growth, follicles allow healthy skin cells to migrate through the skin to help repair damaged tissues. They also allow the skin to release toxins from inside the body. These benefits do come at a price: Follicles are often one of the first areas to show systemic toxicity through acne and folliculitis.

Much like the liver, the kidneys, and the colon, the skin serves the body by absorbing, filtering, processing, and eliminating toxins and excess nutrients from the body. We eliminate toxins through the skin by sweating or through sebum production. Sebum is a fatty substance manufactured by the sebaceous glands. The skin relies on perspiration and sebum to help move toxins through the dermis and out to the epidermis, where they can be shed. Sebum also protects the dermis from dust and debris that can settle into follicles and irritate the skin, and provides a temporary lipid barrier when the skin's existing barrier is compromised.

Both sweat and sebum bring up deposits of crud that our bodies don't want. These deposits can inflame follicles and pores, and cause imbalances in pH levels, oils, and acids. This leads to inflammation, eruption, and scarring. Sometimes this results in acne that does not have excess sebum involved (dry acne). Other times it can simply lead to excess oil production. However, acne mainly erupts as a result of increased sebum, usually due to hormonal influences. Testosterone, which can be elevated in men and women for different reasons, increases sebum production. This, in turn, increases the food supply to bacteria living on our skin. The result is inflammation from the increased bacterial population that leads to redness and swelling. These symptoms are collectively known as acne. Acne occurs most commonly on the face, because our faces contain four to 10 times more sebaceous glands than other areas of the body.

In some instances, the natural processes of perspiration and of sebum excretion may not work well enough to carry away dirt and debris altogether. This is where the pustules and lesions that we know as pimples are actually critical assets to the body's system of self-management. Imagine, if you will, that a piece of dirt has wedged into a pore, accumulated more contaminants and coinciding bacteria, and has begun damaging the skin around it through increased bacterial populations and the effects of the debris. It might be difficult to remove that blockage once it has nestled into our pore, so we need a system that can flush out the follicle. Just as an individual would naturally ask for help moving a couch that is too big and heavy to carry alone, the skin sends out an urgent call for help to relieve the source of inflammation and obstruction in the pore. Enter sebum and immune cells to dismantle the toxins and remove the debris. This often takes a few days to complete. The more toxic the event (high bacteria count or strong irritants), the more likely that the acne lesion will scar. Without the skin's efforts, that debris could make the follicle permanently impaired.

While we are conditioned to regard pimples as unsightly, their very existence is another minor miracle that we should not take for granted. By swelling with pus and sebum, the body has engineered its own solution to the problem of the inflamed pore: The white blood cells, once they reach a critical mass, will burst through the surface of the skin and carry the irritating particles away. While it certainly makes sense to try to calm inflammation—which can be painful, itchy, unsightly, or just plain undesirable—we must remember that the skin is simply doing its job to help eliminate toxins from the body. The key idea in any treatment should be to work with the skin to restore the area with the least amount of additional trauma possible—which is why daily acid therapy is not advised.

CAUSES OF ACNE

To be sure, there is more than one cause of acne. Adolescents develop acne due to a significant testosterone surge during puberty. This testosterone surge increases sebum production, which in turn increases the medium on which bacteria may grow. When bacteria feed off of sebum, their excrement triggers inflammation, which results in the pustules and lesions we commonly identify as acne. Various conditions can cause elevated testosterone levels in both men and women. In fact, a leading cause of acne in women over 30 is an increase in testosterone that usually results from low body-fat levels. Fat cells convert testosterone to estrogen, and low body-fat levels can alter the estrogen-testosterone balance.

Another cause of acne is related to estrogen and progesterone. Women on birth-control pills that raise progesterone levels frequently experience acne as a side effect. Interestingly enough, birth-control pills are also prescribed as an acne *treatment* for women who may not produce enough estrogen to combat the androgens that increase oil production in the skin and block pores, leading to pimples. I raise these points not to discuss pros and cons of birth-control pills but to highlight the roles hormone levels play in the onset and treatment of acne. Our system relies on a precise balance of hormones that is unique for every individual. It can be altered by the foods we eat, by liver toxicity, ovarian cysts, and more. The precise mechanism of how these imbalances affect acne is not clear.

However, scientific research suggests that elevated levels of estrogen and progesterone can result in an increased growth of yeast in the body. Yeast is primarily housed in the digestive tract and may be culpable for as many as 30 percent of the acne cases seen on an annual basis. In addition to cultivating yeast through estrogen and progesterone production, we increase our yeast levels by eating sugar, which provides yeast

> Antibiotics kill harmful bacteria, but they also
> kill healthy bacteria, effectively eliminating
> the "normal flora" (colonized, healthy gut bacteria)
> from our intestines. This creates a ripe environment
> for the spread of *Candida*.

populations with fodder to propagate. This propagation can, in fact, lead to imbalances in the flora (healthy bacteria) that line our digestive tracts. This, in turn, allows for further yeast growth.

How does yeast cause acne? Science doesn't have a definitive answer. Low levels of yeast naturally occur in the intestine and coexist in balance with healthy bacteria as part of the natural order of our internal ecosystems. The most common yeast population among Americans (and this is relevant in part due to diet) is called *Candida albicans*, commonly referred to as Candida. Candida is associated with vaginal yeast infections and thrush (a yeast infection of the mouth and throat). Though it may come as some surprise, these yeast infections actually originate in the intestine. When levels of Candida and bacteria fall out of balance, the yeast emits toxins that travel through the body (via the bloodstream) and result in a variety of physiologic imbalances. My belief is that, if left unchecked, toxic yeast may rise (no pun intended) up and disturb hormone production, impair immune function, and generally wreak havoc on many organs with the skin being a common victim. More than 70 different toxins have been identified thus far, and some of them are hormone mimicking.

Discussion of candida takes an unhappy turn when we consider the common practice of prescribing antibiotics to treat acne. In recent years, American patients (and even their doctors) have begun to ask more questions about the harmful effects of over-prescribing antibiotics. But during the past 30 years, along with the rise of retinoic acid to treat acne and "restore" the skin, antibiotics such as erythromycin, tetracycline, and doxycycline have been widely prescribed to counteract the bacteria that thrive on the sebum our bodies produce every day.

Antibiotics have different effects on our system. Personally, I believe that a significant aspect of their ability to help acne comes from suppressing our immune system. As odd as it may sound, antibiotics are damaging to our immune cells and other cells, which can lead to less inflammation on the skin. Remember, our cells have a tremendous amount of similarity to bacteria and, just as antibiotics have an impact on cell walls or critical cell functions that cause bacteria to die, these yeast toxins impact other cells in the body. Sun sensitivity is common, which is another way of saying that the skin cannot heal very well while on antibiotics. That is not necessarily the right environment for someone who has 50-plus lesions on the edge of scarring. Additionally, antibiotics' effect on digestive health is abysmal and can lead to a variety of concerns. It is not uncommon for an acneic teen given antibiotics to initially see results from the decline in the skin's bacterial population. Yet it is also not uncommon to find that a month or two into the regimen this same teen experiences a bad breakout from the resultant yeast overgrowth. Of course, this flare-up of acne would not be helped by continued antibiotics.

~

The colon is unique in the way toxins build up and solidify along the intestinal wall, creating a cache, if you will, of toxic matter that can leach through the organ and into the bloodstream and, oftentimes, the skin.

~

We've discussed the skin's role in eliminating toxins from the body, and I would be remiss not to discuss another organ, the colon, in the same vein. In my experience, the colon and its related toxin buildup is the primary source of acne. Now, obviously, those toxins don't get there by themselves. We ingest those toxins, generally through food, and our bodies work overtime to rid our systems of the excess baggage. The liver and kidneys also play significant roles in filtering and eliminating toxins. However, the colon is unique in the way toxins build up and solidify along the intestinal wall, creating a cache, if you will, of toxic matter that can leach through the organ and into the bloodstream and oftentimes

Candida Albicans

PHOTO: CDC/DR. WILLIAM KAPLAN

Candida albicans is a single-cell yeast that lives peacefully within the normal ecosystem of our intestines. That is, we've all got some candida on board every day. When the natural flora of our intestinal ecosystem are upset, however, and probiotic bacteria fail to keep the yeast in check, Candida can mutate and becomes a multicellular fungus that, as it grows, presents a very real risk of traveling through the bloodstream to manifest in different parts of the body. In this phase, without intervention, Candida can gradually take over our system, resulting in Candidiasis, a common condition that is underdiagnosed.

In early stages, Candidiasis most commonly presents in the throat, mouth, or vagina, where mucous membranes present a prime environment for colonization. While uncomfortable, this streak of Candidiasis is relatively easy to treat with over-the-counter medications. Systemic Candidiasis presents much more serious problems, especially among sufferers who are already immunocompromised, such as HIV patients or the terminally ill. Systemic Candidiasis presents symptoms ranging from gastrointestinal discomfort, to lethargy, to headaches, to muscle pain. The more we learn about Candida, the more we suspect it as a culprit behind many cases of chronic fatigue, chronic gastrointestinal disorders, and chronic skin conditions.

into the skin. Unfortunately, elimination at this stage is not as simple as just having a good bowel movement. When buildup occurs, the body needs a little help.

I say this because, after years of following various clinics that perform colonics and detoxes, there is no question that client skin improves and acne is significantly diminished upon release of stored toxins in the colon. As such, I firmly believe that we can reduce incidents of acne by promoting colon health through colonics, detoxes, and diet. Ideally, for the ultimate natural elimination of toxins through the colon, I would like to see patients change their diets so they can achieve at least two bowel movements daily. The longer the stool sits in the colon, the more time there is for leaching of these food-derived poisons into our bloodstream.

Just as with the colon, when liver function is compromised—such as through tissue damage resulting from alcohol, medication, or disease— acne may result. A sluggish liver may alter hormone production in an individual, and the resulting hormone levels may trigger oil production and thus acne. Furthermore, a compromised liver will allow more toxins to be released into the bloodstream and the skin, and those toxins block pores, attract bacteria, and lead to acne symptoms.

Finally, acne may be caused by external dirt, debris, and especially chemicals that become trapped in the skin. As we've discussed, the skin is generally adept at a) protecting itself, and b) responding to harmful substances. However, when we meddle with the skin's natural function, all bets are off. Cosmetics that contain ingredients such as isopropyl myristate, for example, can clog pores (comedogenic). When we introduce such chemicals to the skin, we will likely see acne as a result.

ACNE TREATMENTS

It is so much easier to discuss appropriate acne treatments now that we understand in greater detail how the skin functions to remove toxins from the body, and how this normal function can result in acne when all is not balanced within the body's systems. As you'll see, many conventional acne treatments today actually confound the body and work against the skin, as they tackle symptoms without ever addressing the underlying causes of the acne.

What Not to Do

Let's talk a little bit about what we don't want to do when treating acne. As always, we don't want to inflame the skin. We also don't want to dehydrate the skin, which too many skincare products tend to do thanks to their reliance on alcohol, acids, or chemicals. These ingredients function as drying agents designed to strip away oil. Dehydration leads to more fragile skin and a weaker barrier against dirt and debris. As a result, the skin actually produces *more* oil, which worsens acne in many cases.

Remember, by keeping our skin populated with healthy bacteria, we prevent a massive takeover by more harmful bugs.

Skincare products that dehydrate in order to reduce oil succeed only temporarily. As soon as the body senses the imbalance, sebum production spikes in order to protect the skin. It's a perfect catch-22. This is how I believe alpha hydroxy acids create a skin condition referred to as "oily T-zone." The T-zone consists of your forehead and nose, and some of the area around your mouth, including your chin. As you may have guessed, this region is home to a greater number of sebaceous glands than other parts of the face and body. As a result, many people experience more oil, or shine, on this part of their face than they wish to reveal to the world. When I have given these patients barrier-repairing serums, their oily T-zone disappears in days.

Another thing we don't want to do is significantly alter the population of bacteria on our skin, because doing so exposes the skin to a more serious risk of infection. Remember, by keeping our skin populated with healthy bacteria, we prevent a massive takeover by more harmful bugs. The skin is perfectly designed to maintain optimal health when pH levels hover between four and five at the upper level of the epidermis. This pH level provides an ideal environment for the healthy bacteria we want and need. At the same time, the skin's natural acidic barrier reduces the likelihood that unwanted bacteria will flourish on the skin. There are plenty of nontoxic, antibacterial ingredient options that can be used instead of antibiotics and harsh oxidizing chemicals like benzoyl peroxide.

Here's another thing we don't want to do: interfere with the healing of scar tissue. This is a common mistake in treating acne. Much of what we wish to resolve in any acne complaint has to do with appearance. Pimples, and the scars they leave behind, are unsightly. Our focus is usually on the red pimple instead of on the delicate, healing wounds from recent acne lesions. Unfortunately, scar tissue takes a year to heal in most cases. Patients seeking cures for acne are often seeking relief from the active lesions and pay less attention to how the older ones are doing, so they use acids and ignore the delicate, healing areas of the face. Even the active lesions are scarring in front of their eyes and should be treated carefully.

The length of time necessary to allow the body to heal scar tissue is directly at odds with client demand for speedy results. What's more, few of us ever seek help for a single pimple; more likely, an acne sufferer's face or skin is riddled with lesions at various stages of development. It's nearly impossible to apply topical medications to pimples without aggravating healing tissues nearby. In order to restore clarity to the affected areas, we have to get control of the bacterial populations without adding trauma. We must also work on the internal causes. Too many products on the market, however, seek to control bacterial populations topically with wound-impairing irritants. This is where practitioners and the skincare industry have become quite aggressive with salicylic acid, glycolic acid, benzoyl peroxide, and other irritants or inflammatory ingredients. True, such products help control bacteria, but these products also inflame the skin, which leads to a worsening of scar formation. It also leads to a more negative prognosis for the long-term recovery of the affected areas. By triggering inflammation in areas that present scar tissue, we must understand that we are only going to slow the healing process.

Traditional Treatment Approaches

Now that we are familiar with what not to do when treating acne, let's evaluate some common treatment approaches to see how they stack up. If you walk into your local dermatologist's office tomorrow with a complaint of acne, I wager that she'll respond by putting you on a combination of an antibiotic and benzoyl peroxide. Perhaps it will be an antibiotic and salicylic acid. Maybe, if things are really rough or if you've experienced poor results to some previous treatment, the doctor will combine all three in the hopes of stumbling upon an all-chemical solution to your skin woes.

What will happen if you take the dermatologist's advice? I think your symptoms might—*might*—clear up, temporarily. But neither antibiotics nor benzoyl peroxide nor salicylic acid will resolve the underlying problem nor are those options good for the health of the skin. What's more, as we've discussed in fair detail, these solutions will only make your dermatological forecast more gloomy in the long run. The antibiotics will strip the flora from your gut and leave a ripe environment for yeast—the dreaded *Candida albicans*. Benzoyl peroxide and salicylic acid will dehydrate and inflame the skin, and leave it more fragile than before treatment. In response to this insult, your body will push more sebum to the surface specifically to protect the skin, and the cycle will start anew, with oils attracting bacteria and bacteria leading to acne—unless acne had already surged from the Candida.

Another common strategy is to introduce oxygen in some form or another to the surface of the skin. An oxygen strategy includes benzoyl peroxide or hydrogen peroxide, both of which deplete antioxidants and increase inflammation. Remember also that, in Chapter 6, we discussed the perils of the topical application of nutrients—namely, too few of the nutrients penetrate to their target cells. Much of the content of any lotion or cream actually gets lodged in the layers of the epidermis, creating more problems for the skin than it solves. Patients who rely on benzoyl peroxide products often complain of rebound acne. This is because, while the chemical initially controls bacteria on the skin's surface, dehydration, inflammation, and immunosuppression trigger increased sebum production. This, in turn, feeds bad bacteria.

Retinols are another commonly prescribed treatment for acne. Retinoic acid has some effects on clearing acne, but the additional impairments to skin health, including more inflammation and damage to collagen and the barrier, make it less than ideal. Retinoic acid is also not antibacterial. But retinaldehyde, the storage form of retinoic acid and its immediate precursor, has none of the negative effects of the acid while being antibacterial. There are specialized retinols, like Tazorac, that have more-targeted acne effects and are probably safe for the skin. However, I still prefer retinaldehyde over all of them.

Another drug commonly prescribed to attack acne is isotretinoin, which goes by the brand name Accutane. Isotretinoin is tretinoin (retinoic acid) in oral form, and it appears effective in treating acne because is really does reduce oils on the skin, eliminating fodder for bacteria. This makes it extremely popular despite the well-documented fact that it is highly toxic and carries very serious and potentially dangerous side effects. Research is clear that isotretinoin affects everything from mental state—the drug promotes depression and suicidal thoughts—to facial swelling, and can cause organ damage and hinder wound healing because of the intense load the chemicals place on just about every organ in the body. Women who take isotretinoin must not become pregnant while taking the drug—and even shortly after—because of the severe risk of birth defects.

Despite everything we're told about isotretinoin's rejuvenating characteristics, the drug actually interferes with the skin's ability to heal. Not only does isotretinoin result in sun sensitivity, but is also increases aging in a dramatic way due to the intense toll it takes on the tissues of the skin. Obviously, a teenager who is prescribed Accutane is unlikely to think too much about aging, but he should. Adolescence and early adulthood is exactly when the skin undergoes changes that render it less and less capable of tolerating the burdens of daily use. Precisely because isotretinoin impacts the skin's ability to heal, repercussions of the drug's use may be evidenced in the patient for years to come. Unfortunately, there has not yet been significant research on these long-term effects of isotretinoin use.

Two more treatment approaches are worth mentioning. Chemical peels are sometimes administered in the treatment of acne. This is motivated by the belief that the skin needs help exfoliating and the bacteria need to be "nuked." I cannot say enough to dissuade the reader from taking this approach to clearing up acne. Mild peels that interject calming ingredients with nontraumatic antibacterial ingredients are a suitable option for acne, and it does not significantly worsen the likelihood of scarring. Another strategy to control acne is LED light therapy, or "blue light" therapy. LED therapy controls bacteria populations on the skin's surface when sebum production is

> *It's simple, really: Sugar breeds yeast,*
> *and yeast contributes to acne.*

high. This is actually a reasonably effective approach to controlling acne but it does require daily treatments in order to be truly effective. Additionally, there are many lasers that are designed for acneic skin. Some lasers use wavelengths that kill bacteria and can be quite effective. Other lasers are designed to reduce redness, and we discussed those in greater detail in Chapter 3.

Healing Acne from the Inside Out (and, Gently, from the Outside In)

So far, we've covered how acne develops, what not to do when treating it, and common treatment methods (most of which do the things we should actually avoid if we hope to achieve positive, long-term results). Now, let's explore my philosophy on how to treat acne. First and foremost, I encourage you, the reader, to take a good long look at your diet and your digestive history to assess whether you may have toxins built up in the colon. If you've eaten average amounts of non-organic meat, dairy, or produce; eaten large amounts of heavily processed foods or junk foods; taken medications frequently or for long periods of time; or ingested chemicals or synthetics that are hard for the body to eliminate, then you may be overdue for a detox.

At first glance, it may not sound like the most overt treatment for acne, but I strongly recommend assessing your diet to identify opportunities to increase your fiber intake. That's right: Fiber will help lessen your acne symptoms. The more you can encourage the elimination of toxins through the bowels, the less your skin will have to work to pick up the slack. Two healthy bowel movements every day will relieve your skin of a lot of its responsibilities to remove toxins from the organs or bloodstream. Instead, your skin can focus simply on maintaining its own balance and health. To this end, consider an initial series of colonics to jump-start your detoxification process. Then follow up with a colonic once every six months or so, especially if you eat a good deal of dairy.

Look closely at buying and eating organic foods. Too many of the added growth hormones in our meat and dairy end up in our systems, and the body responds with its own hormone shifts. As a result, we see another opportunity for yeast to become dominant in the body, and this contributes to acne. Eating organic produce and avoiding the residual pesticides carried into our bodies through so many conventional fruits and vegetables will allow the immune system to function much more capably. A healthy immune system, in turn, responds more rapidly, more robustly, and more effectively to compromises in the skin that result from irritants.

I also recommend cutting out sugar. Although the dermatological community is of mixed opinion on this matter, I am firm in my conclusion of a yeast-acne link. It's simple, really: Sugar breeds yeast, and yeast contributes to acne. Cut out sugar because, too often, it's an ingredient hidden among many others that causes inflammation. Hydrogenated oils, sodium, and synthetic flavorings all incite inflammation in the body. Just as we must understand and avoid inflammatory agents on the surface of the skin, we must also understand and avoid inflammatory agents taken internally. Inflammation—even internally—stimulates oil production, and oil leads to acne. Additionally, it compromises the overall well-being of your immune system, which leads to problems with wound healing and bacterial control, as well.

A good diet and healthy nutrition provide the foundation for a strong and balanced body, inside of which organs and systems work in harmony to maintain all of the body's needs. I can't say enough about the benefits of a healthy diet in achieving healthy skin. Moving to the skin itself, there are a handful of external approaches that I recommend—in conjunction with the aforementioned dietary considerations—for the effective treatment of acne. My Osmosis skincare line features a peel called Facial Infusion that does not trigger inflammation and helps to control bacteria. It also assists in the removal of toxins and normalizes oil production. It uses high doses of liposomal retinaldehyde, high

*Zinc fingers are proteins at the cellular level that
activate genes and help in the production
of collagen and other cellular proteins.
When used topically, this technology provides
the skin with the tools needed to improve
its overall performance.*

doses of a great anti-inflammatory and antibacterial called liposomal willow herb extract, along with a host of 22 other active ingredients that calm and promote repair in the skin while reducing the bacterial population. I strongly prefer this approach to acid-based peels because it does not add inflammation, it encourages wound repair, and it reduces bacteria counts.

I also believe that LED lights can be effective in controlling bacterial populations. For this reason, light therapy is a welcome addition for clients who have the means and the patience to incorporate it into their daily regimens. Research shows the right light can reduce acne lesions by as much as 85 percent over eight weeks, without additional products.

An option that is admittedly outside the box is Harmonized Water. I am very excited about its potential to help acne sufferers. Harmonized Water is water that has been "frequency enhanced" by imprinting radio waves onto its molecules. These frequencies can have health-promoting benefits on the body. Our cells all vibrate at specific frequencies, and when they are not functioning properly, their vibration shifts. Harmonized Water has the potential to re-establish cellular energetic balance. Our acne clients typically notice a difference in the first month. We also use Harmonized Water topically, in a solution I call Clear, a topical spray that controls bacteria and improves the repair response of the skin.

Another topical approach worthy of strong consideration is the deployment of liposomal retinaldehyde. Liposomal retinaldehyde is unique in the treatment of acne for multiple reasons. First, the liposome itself, phosphatidylcholine, can clear acne by 70 percent on its own. Phosphatidylcholine works to repair the skin's barrier, the epidermis. When the epidermis is healthy and vibrant, moisture levels come into balance and the skin no longer feels the need to produce oil to protect its outermost layers. Less oil means less food for bad bacteria—all thanks to phosphatidylcholine. Couple the liposome with retinaldehyde, and you have a powerful combination because it penetrates better to reach the deep, smoldering inflammation found in acne.

Retinaldehyde is both antibacterial and non-inflammatory. As an ingredient in the treatment of acne, retinaldehyde controls bacterial populations and supports new collagen and elastin formation without creating inflammation in the skin. Additional nutrients can also be delivered via liposome, such as niacinamide, which has been shown to reduce bad bacterial populations, restore the skin's barrier, and promote wound healing.

Topically, tea tree oil is a very effective ingredient against acne, so long as it is used in moderation and in conjunction with other antibacterial ingredients. 1,3 beta-glucan can help promote skin health and control acne. 1,3 beta-glucan triggers a macrophage reaction in the skin, which reduces scarring and reduces bacterial overgrowth. Another noteworthy topical acne fighter is mandelic acid, made from almonds, which, when used in concentrations below five percent, gently controls bacteria without causing inflammation. To complete the strategy, we use liposomal willow herb extract because it has proven anti-inflammatory and anti-bacterial qualities, the perfect combination for acne.

Finally, we know that various clays help to draw toxins out of the skin. As part of a balanced, thoughtful, and logical regimen, clay masks can be used to help the skin eliminate toxins and thus clarify the complexion, especially in cases of acne.

⌒

Inflammation of the digestive lining corresponds
with inflammation of the skin.

⌒

Rosacea

Some 30 million (15 million diagnosed, 15 million not) Americans suffer from rosacea, and that number is continuously growing. Scientists like to blame the sun or immune system failures in the skin for rosacea. They have even blamed Demodex mites—tiny parasitic mites that live in or near hair follicles. To be sure, it makes a certain amount of sense to examine the skin for clues to rosacea's origins, especially because the chief complaint is redness or a network of broken capillaries on the surface of the skin. I don't completely dispute any of these assertions, yet I find a more compelling flashpoint for rosacea well beneath the skin. Like acne, I believe that many of the causes of rosacea occur internally.

One cause of rosacea is *Helicobacter pylori*, a bacterium that can flourish in the stomach, usually as a result of reduced acid production. Another likely cause is Candida and its ill effects on digestion. Additionally, people with ulcerative colitis, Crohn's, and other nebulous digestive issues can often suffer the classic signs of rosacea on the face.

Interestingly enough, I have interviewed several hundred rosacea sufferers over the last few years, and I asked each one of them the following question: Do you have any diagnosed digestive disturbances, or do you have any issues with digestion, including acid reflux, indigestion, constipation, diarrhea, or reactivity to specific foods? Roughly 75 percent of respondents indicated that yes, they did in fact have some associated digestive problem. Consider also another major cause of rosacea—high quantities of alcohol that damage our digestive lining—and you begin to see a pattern clearly emerge: Digestive inflammation corresponds with inflammation of the skin.

As a response to inflammation likely caused internally, the skin increases circulation to an affected area. This vasodilation opens up the blood vessels and deepens the appearance of redness in an already inflamed space. Smoldering inflammation in the skin also renders the body unable to maintain its normal repair and production processes. This results in scar tissue at the site of any damage or inflammation.

Typically, capillaries in the dermis are hidden from view by layers of collagen. This is not the case among later-stage rosacea sufferers. Our skin reflects the inflammation that lingers in our intestine. That secondary inflammation of the skin also results in thinning of the skin. What happens is that the skin cannot maintain appropriate collagen levels. Thinning of the dermis ensues, and capillaries—which are enlarged in response to inflammation—appear through the skin's surface as the "collagen cover" diminishes.

Rosacea treatment, unfortunately, is akin to acne treatment: Doctors usually write prescriptions for antibiotics, which can help the visible signs but fail to resolve the underlying issues. Here's something your dermatologist won't tell you: Even if you take antibiotics, your skin will continue to worsen and decline over the years. Oral antibiotics will cause a further decline in the digestive lining in many cases; therefore I don't recommend that approach. I think that most of the "improvement" topical antibiotics render on rosacea is due to their tendency to suppress inflammation. To be clear, this may make the skin look better but the topical antibiotics are not functioning as an anti-inflammatory. Suppressing immune activity and calming inflammation are two completely different things.

Another common rosacea treatment involves the use of lasers. Laser treatment is a topical response to a handful of visible blood vessels on a patient's cheeks or nose. Of course, it is easy and effective to use a laser to shut down those capillaries and essentially decommission them. This results in an often immediate improvement in the blood vessels that are most visible on the surface of the skin.

But wait—there's a catch. Laser treatment for rosacea strips the skin of blood vessels just when it wants them most—to repair the damage. Remember, adult skin remains in a state of starvation, and the loss of our nutrient delivery can encourage dermal thinning. So what does the skin do in response? It begins building new blood vessels. New capillaries begin forming almost immediately, because the skin believes that it is under siege and must route more resources to the affected areas. The question remains: How much damage occurs while the skin waits for its capillary reinforcements?

My approach to addressing rosacea is somewhat different. First, we must understand the internal conditions before we can effectively treat the external conditions. When treating rosacea sufferers, I strongly

~

One in three women who take "the Pill" experience
some degree of melasma as a side effect.

≈

recommend they take probiotics routinely to promote digestive well-ness. For sufferers with considerably inflamed digestive tracts, I even recommend taking aloe juice (organic) on a daily basis to help soothe the digestive lining. In addition to probiotics and aloe juice, I recommend combining Harmonized Water with Clear Skin and the Digestive Health. Both of these products are designed to reduce rosacea symptoms at the source. Some people with rosacea will even improve with hydrochloric acid supplements and/or digestive enzymes if their issue is compromised digestive juices.

Once we've begun to restore balance internally, it's appropriate to discuss topical rosacea treatment options. Liposomal retinaldehyde, which we discussed in the treatment of acne, is truly one of the best options available to treat rosacea. This is because the liposome itself helps to restore the epidermal barrier. That alone will reduce inflammation significantly—and reduced inflammation means reduced blood surge, which translates to fewer visible blood vessels. What's more, retinaldehyde is the only non-prescription ingredient that has been proven to reduce the symptoms of rosacea.

Liposomal 1,3 beta-glucan is also an appropriate response to rosacea because it improves the skin's repair response and helps alleviate scar tissue that builds up in rosacea sites. Additionally, liposomal willow herb is another anti-inflammatory ingredient that fights unhealthy bacteria and assists the skin's healing processes.

Melasma and Hyperpigmentation

Like rosacea, melasma is a rapidly growing condition in the United States and abroad. It is estimated that one in 15 women in the United States and one in three women in Asia have this incurable affliction. Melasma is a darkening of the skin in response to hormonal changes in the body, specifically the hormones estrogen and progesterone. While melasma presents across lines of sex and ethnicity, it most often appears in pregnant women and women who take oral contraceptives. In fact, one in three women who take birth-control pills experience some degree of melasma as a side effect. While symptoms of melasma generally lessen as hormone levels return to normal post partum, at least one-third of thoses who suffer pregnancy-induced melasma and two-thirds of those who stop birth-control pills have the condition persist indefinitely.

Melasma and hyperpigmentation are related in the following way: If you punch-biopsy a melasma site, you'll find nothing out of the ordinary except for the occurrence of hyperpigmentation or the excess production of melanin in the affected area. We know that melasma is hormone-related hyperpigmentation; additionally, other forms of hyperpigmentation may result from sun damage, scarring, or other prolonged inflammation. Interestingly, melasma responds positively to antifungal medications in many cases, which supports a theory of internal yeast imbalances as an additional cause of melasma. When hormone levels rise, yeast growth increases in the intestine and possibly elsewhere. Pregnancy and birth-control pills both increase hormone levels and likely increase yeast population, which explains why, when the hormone-altering effects are gone, yeast levels and melasma often remain.

Melasma presents a particular challenge to treat topically. Because of its relationship to hormone levels and its sensitivity to the sun, it is often very difficult to treat. First, we need to remove the primary cause, either via the delivery of an infant or the cessation of birth-control pills. Next, the patient needs to use a sunblock like titanium or zinc to reduce the chance of exacerbation.

Topical treatments can be very effective, but most fall way short. Many women have aggressive peels or lasers to lift the pigment temporarily. While I used to offer this service, my experience is that the cost, pain, and suffering—as well as the very temporary results—make those strategies less appealing. Almost without fail, by the next menstrual cycle, the pigmentation has returned. The other possibility is that these traumatic procedures can worsen the area by making it bigger or darker.

With this evidence in mind, I return to the notion that melasma is best treated with a combined topical-internal approach. If we can impact the disturbance in the melanocytes that results in darker pigmentation, and/or if we can eliminate the source of the disturbance in the melanocytes, then we can affect lasting change in the appearance of the skin. To do so, we need to ensure healthy bacteria levels, healthy detoxification and elimination processes, and minimal interference with hormone levels. To be clear, I'm not taking a stand one way or another on birth-control pills. I'm simply saying that, from a skin-first standpoint, we must remove the initial cause if we are to be effective. Antifungals like caprylic acid and prescription medicines have had positive effects on the condition in cases I have witnessed personally.

Once internal balance is restored, there are topical techniques that will assist the skin to correct excess pigment production. Zinc finger technology shows promise in its ability to correct excess melanin production while allowing for normal production to be maintained. This is a major advantage because any therapies that reduce your overall pigment production are going to age you. Zinc finger technology does the opposite, and even offers SPF protection in the process.

The issue with melasma is that patients have to apply lighteners twice daily to have any hope of helping the condition. Additionally, in many cases this becomes a regimen needed for the rest of their lives, so the impact on the skin can be too harsh. Hydroquinone is the gold standard, but it is too inflammatory and long-term use causes more problems than necessary. There are a number of lightening agents that do the job without adding inflammation to the skin: tetrahydrocurcumioids, watercress extract, paper mulberry bark, Sepiwhite, bearberry, alpha-arbutin, and gamma amino butyric acid (GABA), to name a few.

While hyperpigmentation is a symptom of melasma, the two are not always linked. Hyperpigmentation is the excessive production of melanin in specific areas of the skin. While melasma is associated with systemic imbalances, hyperpigmentation itself is primarily the result of local damage. As such, hyperpigmentation is largely isolated from internal causes. In the following paragraphs, I will address three main causes of hyperpigmentation and the various treatment options relevant to each cause.

To understand hyperpigmentation, we must first appreciate the value of our melanin and the cells that make it, called melanocytes. Melanocytes are a critical first-line defense of the skin. They suffer more DNA damage than most other cells in the body because of their location in the epidermis. As soon as we step into the sun, free-radical damage begins. This immediately triggers the production of melanin as the skin adapts to its new environment. Over years of this behavior, melanocytes are beaten up until they are replaced by stem cells that mature into new melanocytes, and then the replacements are beaten up as the process repeats itself throughout our lifetime. While this is true of other cells in the epidermis like keratinocytes, in their case the replacement cells come in every 30 days, whereas melanocytes can last months to years. This is important to understand because it explains why we develop age spots and hopefully helps you to recognize the need to work with them as opposed to treating melanocytes as the enemy. Another way in which age spots develop is through the migration of melanocytes into groups. This bunching effect is understandable because it is meant to protect that area better, but the net result is aesthetically undesirable. The last thing I will mention before we discuss the strategies to help these conditions regards the skin's intelligent design. When we start to get more UV exposure during the sunnier months of spring and summer, our skin has a seasonal adaptation in which it produces more melanin on a regular basis for several months because it knows it faces an uptick in UV exposure then. This may make your spots look worse but it will prevent you from aging faster.

Speaking of intelligent design, the epidermal barrier's unique ability to reflect the majority of light is my recommendation for your first-line defense against hyperpigmentation. This needs to start at an early age. If you avoid exfoliation and UV excesses, there is a much greater likelihood that your melanocytes will be in great shape well into your 50s. Most hyperpigmentation is DNA based, which means that protecting DNA (and repairing it) is an important first step. I understand that this flies in the face of the current wisdom of exfoliating the skin routinely to "help" hyperpigmentation. As we have stated previously, the mild benefits seen with this approach do not justify the long-term negative effects on melanocytes and every other aspect of skin health. Obviously, it makes sense to fortify our skin's natural protective ability with sunblocks (not sunscreens!) like titanium dioxide or zinc oxide.

There are some additional reasons why our skin develops hyperpigmentation that better explain why age spots can be challenging. Research has found that directly below many of these age spots are collections of debris. This suggests that there may be a nutrient-delivery problem. Remember that your melanocytes fire up when free radicals increase—the antioxidant population near the melanocytes provides a natural way to prevent that problem. The debris found may very well interfere with normal antioxidant delivery from the dermis. With fewer antioxidants, the age spot will form wherever the debris resides. Areas adjacent to the spot that have not accumulated debris produce normal melanin levels because they get their normal allotment.

Hyperpigmentation Strategies

LIGHTENING AGENTS

This class of treatment is the gold standard. Hydroquinone leads the group, but as you read in Chapter 4, it is not ideal for skin health. To be fair, all lighteners—ingredients that reduce the amount of melanin in your skin—ultimately speed your skin's aging process by lowering the percentage of one of the few sun-protection strategies the skin has. But hydroquinone adds an additional problem because it damages and inflames the skin. I have found many lightening agents that can function effectively (see list above) without exfoliating or adding inflammation. Lighteners often interfere with the normal production of melanin through a variety of mechanisms, most commonly by interfering with the enzyme tyrosinase, which is a key part of the creation of melanin. The good news is that lighteners often work well and result in significantly less-visible age spots. The bad news is that these lighteners are not corrective and must be used consistently for life. Liposomal delivery of lighteners increases their efficacy by delivering more active ingredients to the deep epidermis, where the melanocytes reside.

EXFOLIANTS

This category includes vitamin C, alpha hydroxy acids like glycolic acid, and a variety of other acids or scrubs designed to speed up the epidermal turnover rate in order to achieve lighter skin. As we discussed above, exfoliation leads to a worsening of hyperpigmentation in the long term. But short term, you may notice that it lightens age spots. This is not corrective; it is a side effect of pushing the epidermis faster than it can handle, thereby reducing the amount of melanin deposited on the skin. I do not recommend this option because it leads to less protective melanin and more free radicals throughout the skin.

ZINC FINGER TECHNOLOGY

This is an exciting new approach to hyperpigmentation because it normalizes melanin but does not shut it down. In other words, it allows the rest of your skin to protect itself and to stay healthy while healing the melanocytes. In fact, evidence has established that this DNA strategy protects the skin to the level of SPF 14.

ACID PEELS

This is another common practice that has some benefit. The idea is simple: If we burn several layers of the epidermis, we will force the skin to rapidly replace itself. This quick action prevents the new skin from getting its full allotment of melanin, which makes everything lighter. If you can figure out how to keep the melanocytes from ramping up again, it is not a bad way to tackle the problem. If not, the benefits are lost over the following weeks as the skin returns to "normal." Two outcomes from acid peels are worth noting. First, it is possible that you have a hyperactive melanocyte (from DNA damage) that the acid destroys. In that case, you may have a more permanent effect on that spot. The second outcome is that the acid inflames the skin and worsens the hyperpigmentation. We cannot control the acid's depth and level of inflammation perfectly, so this occurs on a regular basis.

ANTIOXIDANTS

In general, the delivery of antioxidants from topical products has not proven to be a very effective way to lighten hyperpigmentation. Vitamin

> In the long run, retinoic acid and alpha hydroxy acids do more harm than good. As a result, both the epidermis and dermis are worse off, actually aging faster than if left to their own resources.

C works to a certain degree, but that effect may be related to its exfoliation effects more than free-radical protection. Most topical antioxidants have a tough time reaching the lower epidermis. For that reason, liposomal antioxidants make more sense. But beyond topical antioxidants, the best way to improve your natural protection is by increasing your natural levels. There are two ways to do this: Increase blood flow with ingredients like liposomal niacinamide to feed the skin; and liposomal 1,3 beta-glucan, which triggers the macrophages to come in and remove debris that may be blocking the feeding of that part of the epidermis.

Aging

Finally, we must discuss a skin condition that none of us will avoid: aging. Without a doubt, we will all experience the effects of aging on our skin, and—aside from premature death—there's really no way around the matter. What we can influence, to a large degree, is how quickly our skin ages. There is clear evidence that if you avoid significant sun exposure in your life and your skin maintains healthy antioxidant levels, the signs and symptoms of aging skin will be much less severe.

To be sure, none of us can avoid inflammation for our entire lives. Dealing with inflammation is part and parcel of the skin's role in the body, but inflammation from diet and stress, as well as our tendency to overwhelm the skin on occasion, adds to the skin's challenges. Much of this book is dedicated to avoiding unnecessary inflammation wherever possible, especially in the treatment of inflammation-related skin conditions. One thing we can do to help our skin is to maintain healthy nutrient levels and minimal toxin levels through what we eat. This will help the skin maintain beneficial levels of antioxidants. Those of us who produce higher levels of antioxidants and who remove toxins more effectively will manage inflammation better over the long run than those who don't.

Consider the example of African-American skin. As we've already discussed, African-Americans typically show fewer wrinkles through middle age than do their lighter-skinned counterparts. This is because African-Americans enjoy a natural SPF level of 13.4, thanks to the melanin output in their skin. Their skin is still damaged, but black skin can handle the damage better since it requires less repair. This ultimately prevents significant dermal thinning and the wrinkles that follow.

For those of us who do not enjoy naturally darker skin, there are things we can do to minimize the impact of inflammation over time. Smoking is extremely hard on the skin because it reduces circulation, stimulates cortisol, and exposes the body to many toxins. On a related note, poor dietary habits will manifest in skin stress, as well. Failure to ingest healthful nutrients deprives the skin of much-needed nourishment that allows it to heal. Ingestion of sugars, chemicals, and synthetics will result in the release of cortisol and/or adrenaline, both of which reduce nutrient delivery and hamper repair efforts. Such reactions also accelerate aging. Avoid smoking and eat well in order to help the skin handle inflammation through the years.

Recall that the dermis thins at a rate of 1 percent per year after the age of 20. As we age, we are constantly losing the fibroblasts that produce collagen and elastin. We also lose melanocytes over time, which hastens the aging process. In addition, circulation declines, which leads to a host of skin changes including all of the above-mentioned losses. The combination of these losses with the addition of growing scar tissue and debris is what defines aging in our skin.

Aging skin has some important characteristics that you need to understand. The epidermis does get affected over the long term, even though it is constantly replacing itself. The continued UV damage depletes stem cells for the keratinocytes and melanocytes, and we can see a buildup of the top layer called the stratum corneum. The net result of these losses, plus the decline in its nutrient supply, is why the epidermis slows down and why, over time, it heals more slowly and looks more ragged. Most of these issues are correctable; however, the loss of stem cells is not. This is why we need to give more thought to the ingredients or strategies that deplete our stem-cell supply. There is a variety of changes that occur in the dermis over time. There is a net loss of collagen and elastin as the skin tears down damaged collagen at a faster rate than it makes the replacements. Exfoliation, alpha hydroxy acids, hydrogen peroxide, and retinoic acid cause more damaged collagen. Caffeine, stress, and steroids reduce new collagen formation by decreasing the necessary nutrient supply. When the skin loses its brick-and-mortar structure, the remaining "dermal Jell-O" becomes much more moveable. This is why we see wrinkles.

While the area around the eyes is slightly thinner, the wrinkles around them are from facial expressions. As we sleep, the dermis usually migrates back to being level, which makes our lines worse. As the day wears on, gravity and our facial muscles create new gaps in the dermis. Botox works by stopping the muscles of facial expression, thereby preventing the formation of gaps. We also have a loss of capillaries (and the nutrients they provide), as well as increasing numbers of capillaries that are not fully functional due to damage from UV exposure. The skin cells decline as their DNA shortens. There are also fewer cells as they self-destruct with critical losses to their DNA. Immune activity declines on par with the loss of circulation. Immune repair is further impaired due to excessive exfoliation. The net result is a loss of dermal thickness every year of our adult lives.

Mainstream strategies to treat aging skin primarily rely on peptides, retinols/retinoic acid, vitamin C, and the family of alpha hydroxy acids. Much of their visible effects are the result of exfoliation and plumping, neither of which actually help the skin's aging problem. In the long run, retinoic acid and alpha hydroxy acids do more harm than good. Damage done to the epidermis will always make it impossible for the skin to maintain itself, and it definitely cannot recover losses with the additional trauma and starvation that result. The amount of free radicals that results from a loss of melanin or an exposed barrier is insurmountable. As a result, both the epidermis and dermis are worse off, causing skin to actually age faster than if left to its own resources.

st 10 years of formulating and being active in the aesthetic
, . have been amazed with the exceptional results obtained with
my current philosophy and ingredients. Most of this approach has been
discussed already, but an important part of the success is our ability to
deliver more corrective ingredients into the deeper layers of the skin.
This approach also reduces the breakdown of these delicate ingredients,
along with reducing the sun-sensitizing effects that they create. I also
think it is critical to add nutrient-enhancing ingredients. As we have
identified, niacinamide and 1,3 beta-glucan have positive effects and
allow the fibroblasts to respond to the request for more collagen. Just
telling your skin to make more collagen will not work unless you give
it the tools needed, like amino acids and mineral cofactors. In fact, the
addition of these components topically has proven to be equally if not
more exciting because they create zinc fingers that have the ability to correct several aspects of aged skin.

In the preceding paragraphs, we've considered the facts and reviewed
some traditional approaches. At the end of the day, the best ways to
counteract the effects of aging are to 1) protect the skin's barrier to minimize the workload of the skin, 2) maintain healthy nutrition topically
and internally to give the skin the opportunity to thrive, 3) use targeted
liposomal therapy to restore skin cells at all levels of the skin, and 4)
use zinc finger technology to repair damaged DNA. While other treatments may offer short-term benefits, no other treatments that we know
of today can do as much for the skin.

To Review

We've covered a lot of ground in this chapter. My hope is that, after considering basic conditions within our bodies and studying some of the
more common skin afflictions and their respective treatments—both
guided and misguided—the reader will have a finer appreciation for how
truly basic the underlying principles of skin health can be. In that light,
a few takeaway ideas become clear.

Always consider that what we put into our bodies must find a way out.
We can make the process of elimination easier on our organs, including
the skin, by eating with care. By avoiding toxic buildup in the bowel, we

By trusting in our bodies to know how to self-manage, and by working with the body when it needs a little help, we can alleviate a great number of the conditions and complaints described here.

also avoid long-term strain on the body as our various systems attempt to dispose of toxins. The skin is an organ of detoxification in the same way that the liver, intestine, and kidneys are organs of detoxification. The easier we make it on the skin, the longer it will be able to maintain health and balance on its own, without intervention.

The importance of eating healthfully to improve skin nutrition and function becomes even more apparent as we look at acne, rosacea, and melasma. While each of these conditions manifests in and on the skin, my argument is that each of them likewise is rooted in internal factors. Yeast, the noted *Candida albicans*, must be kept in check if we are to be systemically healthy. To this end, healthy bacteria levels are critical. We maintain healthy bacteria in our systems by maintaining healthy hormone levels. While each of us will experience hormonal shifts throughout our lives, many common treatments for our skin complaints either eradicate probiotic bacteria or result in hormone imbalances (which also sways the balance of probiotic bacteria).

Yeast feeds on sugar, so cutting out sugar is one of the best dietary decisions we can make. Likewise, foods that inflame the intestine will also inflame the skin. In addition to curtailing sugar consumption, we should avoid chemicals and preservatives our bodies were never meant to digest. Alcohol is extremely inflammatory, which gives us another good reason to enjoy it in moderation.

Keep in mind that, although we find pimples unappealing, the pus behind each zit is actually our body's emergency-response team to the rescue. The accumulation of white blood cells represents an outstanding effort to remove unwanted irritants from the surface of the skin. Any intervention that we take must complement, not suppress, the body's innate dermatological response. Understand also that scar tissue takes a year to heal in most cases. Applications of retinoic acid and alpha hydroxy acids inflame the skin. While these medications may reduce bacteria populations, they also slow the healing process of existing scar tissue. As we mentioned earlier, few acne sufferers have the pleasure of battling one pimple at a time. More often, active lesions appear near healing wounds, so the acids that battle bacteria on the new pimple are damaging the delicate and sensitive site of the old one.

Relative to acne, antibiotics are not a sustainable and healthful long-term solution for the skin. While antibiotics do control bad bacteria on the skin, they also destroy the good bacteria that keep yeast in check. Long-term antibiotic users open themselves up to intense immunosuppression, and, on top of that, create an environment in which yeast may thrive. Isotretinoin, another popular acne treatment (commonly known as Accutane), presents one of the greatest successes in the treatment of acne but does so at the greatest of costs. The side effects are, without exaggeration, life threatening. Benefits of isotretinoin and any strong medication must be weighed against the potential harm they present. In this case, the risks outweigh the benefits. What's more, the entire tretinoin family does more to accelerate skin deterioration over time than to restore overall skin health.

Rosacea sufferers may take heart that, by reducing inflammatory foods and through application of liposomal retinaldehyde and zinc finger technology, we now have promising ways to decrease the appearance of those spider webs of capillaries on our skin. Always remember that exfoliation is rarely, even by the most cavalier of practitioners, mentioned in conjunction with rosacea. Instead, antibiotics and steroids are the most common first line of defense, followed closely by laser treatments to decommission over-dilated blood vessels. My advice to the rosacea sufferer is to first seek recourse internally. Once internal inflammation is reduced, liposomal delivery of retinaldehyde and zinc finger components can significantly repair cells damaged by rosacea.

Melasma and hyperpigmentation, while not painful, may still cause distress because of their impact on appearance. Melasma, remember, is a hormone-related condition common among women taking oral contraceptives or during pregnancy. While melasma occurs because of internal shifts in hormone levels, its chief symptom, hyperpigmentation, presents in the skin. For treatment of melasma, we must restore healthy hormone levels and control yeast. Only then can we execute non-inflammatory lightening therapies to restore even skin tone.

Hyperpigmentation is unique among the maladies we've discussed because, by itself, there is no known internal component to address in the treatment of the condition. Hyperpigmentation is an extremely localized response to cellular damage, usually connected to UV radiation. Whether it be DNA damage or melanocyte bunching, the skin produces extra melanin that creates noticeable spots on the skin. Our focus should be on cell repair and skin protection first, followed by the use of lighteners and zinc-finger technology. The key is to not add inflammation that will create more spots or worsen existing ones.

Eventually, we will all fall prey to the symptoms of skin aging. To protect against the ravages of time, we should eat healthfully, promote healthy circulation, and work with the skin in its natural repair processes. This means that we should not exfoliate for exfoliation's sake. Nor should we use retinoic acid in the hopes of "rejuvenating" the skin. Both of these represent clear cases of causing more harm than good by creating unnecessary inflammation. It is so much easier to protect and maintain the skin than it is to replace or repair lost or damaged cells.

All in all, common-sense approaches can repel the symptoms of some fairly common skin conditions. My hope is that, by creating an environment in which we discuss the skin in the context of the entire body, we can reduce and perhaps, from individual to individual, eliminate the incidents of skin irritation that cause discomfort or even distress. Most of all, I hope that we can gradually suspend the excessive use of treatments—namely exfoliation, antibiotics, steroids, and skin-impairing ingredients like retinoic acid. By trusting our bodies to know how to self-manage and by working with the body when it needs a little help, we can alleviate a great number of the conditions and complaints described here.

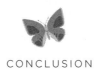

Fixing Problem Skin— for Good

THE SKIN IS ONE of the most fantastically complex and remarkably effective organs in the body. It is self-healing and will continue to renew and repair itself if we refrain from interfering with its normal functions. But for decades, we've been hindering the skin's natural intelligence by slathering on so-called antiaging moisturizers and scrubbing our faces raw with exfoliators that promise to renew the skin. In actuality, the majority of popular skincare products and therapies damage the skin and accelerate its aging, rather than delivering the antiaging and health benefits they promise.

There are tons of scrubs on the market today that are filled with natural ingredients like seeds, beans, and nuts that make them seem safe for the skin. The cosmetics industry has led us to believe we need to slough off the dead skin—so we do, often daily. But the reality is that, as part of its perfectly designed self-renewal system, the skin will shed cells on its own, when it's ready. It doesn't need the help of a treatment that does more harm than good. And what about cleaning up all that dirt that must be clogging the pores and causing pimples? It turns out that our self-healing skin is designed to handle some dirt without developing any complications or infections. I believe that a little dirt is actually healthier for your skin than over-cleansing because of the damage done to the barrier that we discussed.

In this book, I also debunked the belief among skincare professionals that the "dead cells" at the very surface of the skin are responsible for wrinkles, uneven skin tone, and dull, lifeless skin. In fact, those so-called dead cells actually can prevent aging, infection, dehydration, wrinkles, and uneven skin tone, so they should not be forced off with harsh exfoliants and peels. In addition, this top skin layer reflects 80 percent of damaging UV radiation, so when we exfoliate, we leave ourselves open to more UV damage.

Another new concept I hope you accept is that over-cleansing and exfoliating regularly with drug-store scrubs, alpha hydroxy acids, Retin-A®, chemical peels, or dermabrasion treatments can cause far more inflammation than if you had just left the skin alone. When we inflame the skin daily for temporary results, the long-term consequences are actually worse. All of these exfoliation treatments increase inflammation—and anything that induces inflammation should be avoided because it will only exacerbate whatever conditions we are already suffering from, interfere with normal skin health, increase the risk of skin cancer, and lead to more rapid aging.

We are under the mistaken impression that exfoliation speeds up our epidermal turnover rate to what it was when we were young, bringing with it the skin of a 20-year-old. But these results are only temporary, and such traumatic treatments cause age-accelerating inflammation and damage the epidermal barrier.

If you're not convinced that you must end your exfoliation addiction, just look at the overall results of the last three decades of quick-fix chemical peels, laser treatments, exfoliants, microdermabrasion, and youth-promising serums. All of these treatments and products only temporarily plump the skin, lessening the appearance of wrinkles and reducing color to the skin—but at the same time increasing free-radical damage, reducing our sun-protective melanin, and starving the skin of the nutrients and cellular components it needs to maintain its health. Unfortunately, Americans continue to pay for these procedures and creams because they see immediate results. But we don't realize that the effects will not be long-term. This instant improvement in appearance results from plumping of the skin, which is almost always localized swelling that's the result of skin-damaging inflammation. These last 30 years have not made our skin younger, healthier, or more beautiful. Instead, we have seen increases in the prevalence of most skin conditions, including skin cancer.

Think about it. Do the Hollywood celebrities who brag in magazines about these trendy treatments look any younger or better than before they became addicted to such harsh skin therapies? Frankly, I think that the opposite is true. As I look at the skin of people who receive frequent chemical peels, daily or weekly exfoliation treatments, or daily retinoic acid, their skin is thinner and more fragile.

I hope I've convinced you that these procedures are so damaging to the skin that they must be avoided. But even more pervasive are the harmful ingredients in skincare products. In addition to the inflammation-inducing acids like alpha hydroxy acids and retinoic acid, there are other ingredients to avoid, such as parabens, which studies show are linked to serious health risks like breast cancer. Other ingredients to pitch from your makeup bag include sodium lauryl sulfate, glycols, ceramides, and hydroquinone. Also, don't turn to steroids to control inflammation, because that can lead to more skin trauma. Antibiotics are also commonly prescribed to treat rosacea and acne, but their use can compromise your digestive system. And avoid topical oxygen therapy because it generates free radicals in the epidermis, a main cause of skin aging.

What really seems to lead to aging more than anything is sustaining significant inflammatory damage to the skin. This could come in the form of an inflammation-causing treatment or a bad sunburn. For decades, dermatologists have warned us to either avoid the sun or slather on chemical sunscreens any time its rays hit our bare skin. But recent research questions this approach because blocking sun exposure leads to a lack of vitamin D. This increases the risk of many serious diseases. Also, the sunscreens we apply every day may not be effective as we thought at protecting us from harmful rays. Even more concerning, some sunscreens contain toxic chemicals linked to cancer, hormone disruption, allergies, and dermatitis. It's disturbing to realize that the sunscreens we've been religiously applying not only don't seem to be working—they are actually causing harm. But because these chemicals damage DNA, create inflammation, and weaken your immune system, the very thing you're applying to stave off skin cancer could be increasing your risk of the disease.

Along with increases in skin cancer around the world, we are also seeing a rise in skin conditions such as rosacea, melasma, eczema, and psoriasis. I do believe the common skincare approach of regular exfoliation—a treatment known to increase inflammation—contributes to the higher incidence of these troublesome conditions.

Because the skin is constantly inflamed and trying to work out its repair issues, it has a tremendous number of challenges to deal with. The most important challenge is the skin's lack of nutrients. Our skin suffers from the foods we eat and the stress we endure, depleting us of antioxidants and other protective and repairing nutrients. To keep your skin healthy, you must eat nutritious foods and keep your digestive system functioning properly. However, many of us eat processed foods filled with toxic chemicals that do not nourish our bodies. Instead, they cause irritation and inflammation in the digestive tract, impeding its vital function. If you commit to changing your eating habits, you can clear up skin problems.

Turning It Around

Now that you understand that you have problem skin, you can start the healing process. Contrary to the common viewpoint that the skin needs assistance, the reality is that our skin is fighting the good fight 24 hours a day, seven days a week. The last thing it needs is outside interference in the form of inflammation-causing treatments. With that being said, you certainly want to maximize the skin's potential and increase the level of collagen activity, DNA repair, antioxidant production, immune support, and antibacterial action, among other skin activities. The way you can do this is with the ingredients that the skin recognizes and ingredients that the skin can put to better use. That is typically why I choose natural ingredients in my formulas. I think those have the best shot of being utilized within our skin's cells—as long as there is research proving their efficacy.

I believe that the process of promoting skin health starts at the top. Since the skin puts all that time and effort into making your barrier as complete as possible, it only makes sense that we try to maintain that barrier by not exfoliating on a daily basis. You must remember that the skin does not age at the epidermal level, but at the dermal level, so you need to focus attention on strategies like liposomal technology or other approaches that will reach the dermis more effectively. This approach works on two levels. Firstly, by reaching the dermis, we are targeting the right area of the skin since that's where most of the skin issues stem from. Secondly, this approach prevents the ingredients that often can be a source of inflammation or irritation from becoming trapped in the epidermis.

The next step is to stimulate collagen activity. My philosophy at Osmosis is to never create inflammation when boosting collagen production. As I have mentioned previously, when you use glycolic acid to stimulate collagen, you are simply stimulating collagen for the wound that was created by glycolic acid and not for the wounds created by your 30 or 40 years of sun exposure. So we use a lot of fibroblast stimulators, including retinaldehyde, chlorella, GHK copper peptides, epidermal growth factor, niacinamide, 1, 3 beta-glucan, R-lipoic acid, and L-ascorbic acid.

Next, you want to focus your attention on the level of scar tissue that is within the skin. Macrophages within the skin can scavenge and help remove scar tissue and bacteria in the skin. 1,3 beta-glucan does a great job of recruiting more macrophages in your skin.

The final piece of the healthy-skin action plan: repairing DNA. Using zinc finger technology—which also boasts a proven SPF of 14—we have seen evidence of true cellular repair that can improve the aesthetics of facial capillaries, hyperpigmentation, and other skin concerns. We use zinc finger technology to work on the cellular level, repairing damaged cells and improving melanin production.

As you rethink your approach to skin health, keep in mind that, despite our repeated attacks on the skin, this wondrous organ still manages to do a remarkably good job at maintaining itself. Just look past the widely accepted but outmoded skincare therapies that are causing harm and be open to this new approach that helps your skin from the inside out. By trusting your body to know how to self-manage, and by working with your body when it needs a little help, you can alleviate a great number of skin problems and stop the rapid aging that conventional treatments cause. I assure you that you can repair your skin in ways that are healthy and nourishing, not damaging.

Top 50 Skin Questions Answered

Q Should I use sun protection?

A Sometimes. Use sun protection if you are going to be exposed to the sun for more than a total of 20 minutes per day. Do not use chemical or water-resistant sunscreens. Look for all-natural, mineral-based products containing zinc, preferably silica-coated zinc or zinc finger technology, but try to avoid titanium dioxide because some research links it to health risks. Do not sunbathe for any extended period of time. It's not necessary to use sunscreen with a sun protection factor (SPF) higher than SPF 30. Use products offering Harmonized Water protection. Also try wearing clothing that offers protection from the sun's harmful rays.

Q Should I use retinoic acid?

A No. I know that may come as a shock to some, but our skin is not designed to have excess retinoic acid lying around. We do not store retinoic acid, which means our skin struggles to remove the excess. While retinoic acid is proven to stimulate collagen, it also exfoliates and damages collagen in the process.

Q Are moisturizers good for my skin?

A Not often. While restoring skin lipids (with the exception of ceramides) is sun protective and barrier restoring, oil in general is clogging to the skin and moderately negative in its effect on the overall health of the skin. Oil is very susceptible to oxidation, which can lead to the incorporation of oxidized lipids into our cellular structures. Most moisturizers are water-based and contain some oil along with emulsifiers, which are not barrier protective because they make the barrier more permeable. Emulsifiers also are not effective at retaining moisture. Since they often contain ingredients that increase inflammation, they should usually be avoided. Instead, restore moisture the old-fashion way—by not exfoliating it.

Q Should I exfoliate daily?

A No. Exfoliation increases dehydration, aging, and your risk for skin cancer. It also reduces the amount of nutrients your skin has to maintain and fix itself. Remember, your skin already has an exfoliation schedule based on what it is capable of managing, so the best way to improve turnover is to feed the skin.

Q Is my skin starving?

A If you are older than 30, most likely. Every year of our adult life, we lose a little more of our skin's circulation, which is also our skin's sole source of nutrition. The skin slows down its turnover rate when it detects the shortage. Add to that the lack of quality, mineral-rich foods in our diet, and the problem worsens. Finally, consider the deleterious effects to our system of smoking, caffeine, and cortisol, all of which reduce the delivery of skin nutrients. The best way to avoid skin starvation is to increase circulation and protect (not exfoliate) the skin from further inflammation whenever possible.

Q Is it OK to exfoliate once a month?

A Probably. Once a month does not elevate the daily levels of inflammation and will likely not overtax the system. Exfoliation is acceptable when it is associated with other benefits like dermal repair. Don't just exfoliate for the sake of it.

Q How do I keep my skin moist?

A Avoid hot showers, over-cleansing the face, and daily exfoliation because all of those approaches remove the lipids that keep in moisture. Don't count on moisturizers to work unless they have skin lipids in the formula at high doses. And remember to drink plenty of water.

Q Should I use a scrub (or scrub device) on my skin?

A No. Your skin spends a long time (roughly 30 days) making the barrier you have perfect and protective. Why would you want to damage it when you know that scrubbing off the stratum corneum increases aging and your risk for skin cancer?

Q Do lasers make your skin healthier?

A Sometimes, but not usually. That is not to say they don't make your skin look better, because they can certainly do that. However, the question was whether or not they make the skin healthier. Consumers have resigned themselves to the fact that most laser results are temporary, but that did not stop them from having over 10 million procedures last year. Obviously, the vote is in: The temporary results can be worth the money. Just remember that the effects of heat damage (caused by most lasers) are swelling and contraction from tissue loss, not tissue rebuilding and rejuvenation. Lasers can close vascular abnormalities, break up scar tissue, puncture fat cells, and offer other benefits, but the closure of several facial capillaries or the heat damage of collagen are not good for the general health of the skin.

Q Should I use Botox?

A In some cases, it may be worth the risk. First, let's start with the risk. You are putting a neurotoxin into your tissue that may not remain local. This means it may ultimately damage neurons elsewhere in the body, like the brain. Frequent injections can cause hardened, raised bumps of scar tissue, so consider coming at it from different angles with repeated visits. You can bruise for several days, or your eye can become droopy for a few months. The advantage of Botox is that it can stop the displacement of your collagen by keeping your muscles from separating the thinned collagen matrix in your dermis. When these wrinkles are located around the eyes, between the brows, or on the forehead, they are often the result of movement of the gelatinous-like dermal matrix due to less collagen—and that means less structural rigidity. I primarily only recommend the forehead and glabella (between the brows) because Botox around the eyes makes people look funny. That is why we are seeing an increase in the number of people who ask about using less Botox so their face is not completely immobilized. Most of the "top 50 most beautiful people" have become less beautiful, in my opinion, because of their use of Botox. They are wrinkle-free, but they have zombie eyes.

Q Should I use fillers?

A The only filler that makes a great deal of sense to me is hyaluronic acid. It is non-inflammatory (after the injections) and it can temporarily improve density in the dermis. The problem is the cost per month for something that does not work to reverse aging. I think it's time we compare the price per procedure to the true rejuvenation benefits that result.

Q Organic or natural?

A Either one is great in most cases, unless you are looking for real results. I think the growth of organic skincare will wane over the next decade as people realize the organic and corrective cannot coexist with the current labeling laws in place. This has more to do with the current regulations for labeling than the idea of using ingredients from organic plants. If we could get our vitamin C from an organic orange or an antioxidant straight from organic fruit extraction, that would be great. Unfortunately, organic products are so limited in what actives they can contain, they rarely make significant change in the skin. Natural products have a similar problem. We cannot harvest our ingredients from fruits and vegetables in most cases due to the prohibitive costs. That would be the true definition of natural, in my mind. Instead, 99.99 percent of the companies use "bioidentical" active ingredients, which I think are about 90 percent as good as the real thing. There are cases where we would define "natural" much more strictly than it is being claimed. A natural product should not have inflammatory or toxic preservatives like parabens or phenoxyethanol. It should not contain dyes, artificial fragrance, or fillers.

Q Is mineral makeup better than traditional makeup?

A It is in most cases. Most makeup, including foundations, concealers, eye shadows, and lipsticks contain ingredients that are inflammatory. The advantage of mineral makeup is that the ingredients are healthier on the skin and usually sun protective, as well.

Q Is mineral makeup safe?

A Yes, but there are some risk factors. If you inhale a lot of mineral powder during applications, you can cause lung fibrosis if there is uncoated mica or titanium in your makeup. Dimethicone-coated mica prevents the lungs from reacting to it. However, I prefer zinc on the skin over titanium because it helps the skin heal. Once on the skin, zinc can cause mild irritation, especially when sweat moistens the powder, resulting in elevated levels of mineral in the skin. Any mineral can be a source of irritation if it's not supposed to be in the skin. For example, bismuth oxychloride has the potential to irritate if used in excess just like any of the other minerals. If these minerals get past the protective barrier and/or get wet, then mild irritation can be expected. These effects are mild and benign compared to the potential toxins found in traditional makeup, such as copolymers, propylene glycol, and DEA/TEA.

Q Is glycolic acid bad?

A I'm sure glycolic acid serves a purpose in our body. It can be digested and used in some way in the body, just not for the skin. However, people forget that glycolic acid—and most of the other alpha hydroxy acids—don't have receptors in the skin. Glycolic acid works by damaging skin layers, which forces epidermal-barrier repair. That results in fewer nutrients in the dermis. It also causes a loss of lipids, which promotes dehydration and free radicals, increasing aging of the skin and skin cancer risk.

Q Is SPF 50 better than SPF 30?

A No. First, it is unnecessary to have a sun-protection factor (SPF) of 50 because it offers such a minute amount of improved protection from UV rays compared to SPF 30 (SPF 50 provides 99 percent protection, while SPF 30 offers 98 percent). SPF 50 is actually worse than SPF 30 because it adds more inflammation to the skin if you use artificial sunscreens. What has convinced me of this risk is that, since we have been using these UVB-blocking chemicals, all forms of skin cancer have dramatically increased. In addition, a recent study showed that the use of these sunscreens significantly increases the amount of inflammation in our skin. We also are not designed for them. When zinc oxidizes, our skin knows what to do. When a chemical like benzophenone or PABA becomes a free radical, the skin's immune system has to be somewhat bewildered by the odd nature of this ingredient and likely has difficulty protecting against it. Finally, the near doubling of these toxins that is required to jump from SPF 30 to SPF 50 will only further traumatize the skin.

Q What causes puffiness under the eyes?

A It can be genetic or can result with age as we deposit toxins in the fat cells under our eyes. Traditional Chinese medicine says it also relates to kidney disturbances. I think it is a collection of toxins that accumulate in these fat cells. This is why they should be treated with ingredients that increase circulation and immune support rather than decrease it with vitamin K or caffeine-like vasoconstrictors whose common usage further thins and ages the skin in those areas. You can move much of the swelling out over several months through improved circulation and some lipolysis-stimulating ingredients.

Q Why does my skin look dull?

A Dull skin is a sign of immunosuppressed skin. I say that because it implies there is reduced repair activity going on. After all, the more action in the skin, the more circulation (rosiness) can be expected. It may also mean that the skin has reduced melanin activity. Healthy skin never looks dull.

Q Is benzoyl peroxide good for the skin?

A No. While there is a mild reduction in bacteria (assuming the person has an overgrowth of bacteria), benzoyl peroxide interferes with wound healing and depletes antioxidants. This ages the skin and increases scar potential.

Q Is a little Accutane OK?

A No. Sometimes we like to think that a little bit of a toxic substance is not harmful. Would you sweeten your cereal with a little rat poison every day? Accutane (Isotretinoin) is damaging to several organ systems, including the skin. It inhibits normal repair for months, if not years. Although it is not discussed, I am convinced that Accutane rapidly speeds aging in the skin since it has effects similar to steroids.

Q Why am I burning more in the sun?

A Have you noticed that the sun seems hotter and more damaging these days? Whether it is solar flares or ozone depletion or something yet unidentified, we need to be careful. Since we want to get as much healthy sun as possible, we need to maximize the health of the skin so that it tolerates an extended exposure to the sun without long-term ill effects.

Q What are those bumps on my kids' arms?

A Those goose bumps are what are known as keratosis pilaris. I believe they are related to digestion. Exfoliation helps a little, but internal options like Harmonized Water, probiotics, and/or anti-fungals may be more beneficial. The skin on the back of the arm is sensitive, which is why aggressive topical remedies are not well tolerated.

Q How often should I do a chemical peel?

A The classic chemical peel uses an acid to burn the skin to varying depths. Gentle peels either use gentler acids, more-alkaline solutions, or peels that are more superficial due to their larger molecular size. They remove several layers of stratum corneum and the lipids that help hold these layers in place. The benefit is that this peel inflames the skin enough to swell the epidermis and make your fine lines look better, as well as offering a polished, rosy look. It is not rejuvenating by any physiologic measure. Any increase in collagen is clearly being made to repair the superficial damage. Medium-depth peels burn the skin down into the dermis. In this case, they often damage the entire epidermis, including the stem cells, the melanocytes, and the papillary dermis. To be clear, these areas are not particularly old or damaged in most cases. Their replacement cells will probably not be as healthy or efficient as the ones that were burned but they may be less discolored. Damage to the papillary dermis might force some improvement of the organization of the collagen as the skin is forced to lay down replacement collagen. It does not, however, add to the amount of collagen. In some cases, it can result in a loss of collagen. The side benefits of this peel (usually called a TCA peel) is a less discolored epidermis, swelling that minimizes fine lines, and tightening during the wound-healing process. In both peel depths, the side benefits disappear once the skin has finished healing. Repeated peels do not lengthen the time of the side benefits nor is there any incremental improvement in the skin's overall health. Superficial peels can be done monthly without significantly advancing aging. Medium-depth peels may need to be separated by as much as six months to give the skin time to recover. It is possible to speed aging with this type of peel.

Q Is it a good idea to poke holes in the face?

A There has been an increase in the use of devices that essentially "aerate" the skin. It looks better afterward because of the creation of numerous little pockets of inflammation that swell the skin. There is a temporary improvement in fine lines and product penetration, but the added inflammation means aeration will likely not create a net benefit to the skin. In some cases, it can break up scar tissue and possibly help acne scarring.

Q Can aging skin be reversed?

A I am of the belief that the skin will return to its most ideal state if there has not been scarring and if it is given high levels of the nutrients it relies on to function optimally, and it is not continually beaten down by ongoing inflammation. This means you cannot use irritants, you cannot exfoliate, you cannot get sunburns. You must increase circulation and maximize non-traumatic ingredients that encourage the skin to live up to its potential. We must also increase our immune efforts to repair and remove scar tissue. This is best done by activating macrophages. Finally, we need to make repairs at the cellular level to the actual damaged DNA until we can achieve production levels of antioxidants and enzymes that match the skin of our youth.

Q Why do I break out during my period?

A Fluctuations in hormone levels, including the rise of estrogen and progesterone during the latter half of the menstrual cycle, can cause an increase in the conversion of estrogen to testosterone. Testosterone causes an increase of sebum, which feeds the growth of bacteria like *Propionibacterium* acnes. I believe, however, that the majority of breakouts related to menstruation are fungal. The increase in female hormones increases the growth of yeast cells, which are known to cause acne breakouts.

Q Are "liver spots" really from the liver?

A Possibly. There are some hyperpigmented spots that are much more resistant to treatment. Often when we are able to lighten them, underneath is an inflamed spot that never seems to heal. Whether or not there is a relationship with liver damage remains unknown, but those spots behave differently than most age spots.

Q Why do I get facial hair?

A There are two components to facial hair: your genetic makeup and the influence of testosterone. Certain ethnicities have higher levels of villous hair activity. Other women are affected by ovarian cysts, low body-fat levels, and the effects of hormone-laced dairy products.

Q Why am I getting acne after age 30?

A This could be from ovarian cysts. It could be poor elimination and a need for more regularity. It could be elevated yeast levels. It could be a sluggish liver. It could also be from a buildup of a particular toxin.

Q What causes capillaries to show on the skin?

A As the skin loses its dermis at a rate of about 1 percent per year, it eventually thins enough to expose some of the capillaries that are coursing through the dermal layer. This is the most common reason capillaries start appearing. Alternatively, there is some evidence that

DNA damage can send the wrong signals that create unnecessary branches off the capillary bed. Neither of these causes address the more prevalent concern of dilation of these vessels, which is commonly associated with rosacea.

Q What causes spider veins?

A Pressure. It is the current wisdom that spider veins are the result of increased pressure on the venous return to the heart. Pressure can come from bloating, collapse of the supporting structures of our veins, or simply pressure from constantly standing. I am researching the possibility of there being a DNA component since the collections of vessels often show up in areas with fat accumulation, which means the area is exposed to a lot of toxins.

Q Why is my skin dry?

A Americans are about 20 percent dehydrated normally, so it will help to address that problem first. Secondly, the skin cannot hold onto water well if you over-cleanse your face or use exfoliants or exfoliating devices. Essentially, anything that removes parts of your protective barrier is going to allow the loss of hydration to occur.

Q Why does my skin hurt in the sun?

A This is an indication that your skin is not managing sun damage well. It happens to most people when they attempt to go back into the sun—after sustaining a sunburn—within a day or two of the initial exposure. It happens to others almost immediately after exposure. What this indicates is a lack of antioxidants within the skin. Remember, your skin should have the ability to handle 10 to 30 minutes in the sun without developing a sunburn (depending on melanin levels)—not because there is not damage but rather because the damage is managed by our immune system. In summary, pain with sun exposure is your skin's way of sending a warning signal that you are being affected by that UV exposure.

Q Should I use hydroquinone?

A I would not recommend it. Hydroquinone is outlawed in several countries because of its known toxic effects. I have found alternative lighteners, including zinc finger technology, that are safer and more effective. Hydroquinone causes exogenous ochronosis, which is a permanent deposit of pigment in your dermis that is very difficult to treat. It happens in over 65 percent of users according to one study out of South Africa. Hydroquinone also damages your melanocytes, which may cause the long-term consequence of depleting the stem-cell population that replaces melanocytes. Remember, melanocytes are one of our main wrinkle preventers. What I like most about using zinc finger technology is that it normalizes pigment production without stopping its protective benefits.

Q What causes melasma?

A Officially, we do not know, but in my opinion, it is likely liver- or yeast-related issues. We know that certain hormonal levels rise in pregnant women, those who use hormone-replacement therapy, and those who take birth-control pills. It is also a fact that elevated estrogen and progesterone can lead to overgrowth of candida and other fungi. Based on a fungal-looking pattern melasma has on the skin, the likelihood that increased hormones fuel yeast growth in the body, and the fact that the skin often maintains melasma even after the hormone imbalance has been removed, it is reasonable to assume there is a correlation. In case that is a contributor, I recommend anti-fungals to everyone. I also recommend liver cleanses in case patients have suffered damage from hormonal supplementation.

Q Does collagen as an ingredient help the skin?

A Not really. Your skin is not going to incorporate the collagen of a cow or pig into its matrix (nor would I want that!). The effects are from superficial plumping that results from the proteins being trapped in the epidermis. It is generally not worth the money since the results are temporary.

Q What is beneficial about putting caviar on the skin?

A Nothing, really. There may be some minerals that can be utilized but, for the most part, there is a mild plumping effect and not much else.

skin be both dry and oily?

ict, this condition is extremely common. Exfoliation and
nsing will dry out the skin. To protect itself, the skin starts
ig sebum for temporary lipid relief. Areas that have more
sebaceous activity, like the nose, will increase production, causing
the combined event of oil and dehydration.

Q Why do we get rosacea?

A There are a lot of theories. I believe the number-one cause is a digestive imbalance that could be from a yeast overgrowth, *Heliobacter
pylori* infection, inflammatory bowel disease, or something else.
That is why there has been such an increase in cases that correlate
with the increase in digestive issues.

Q Is vitamin C good for my skin?

A Yes. But like everything else, there is a point at which you can have
too much of a good thing. Vitamin C works in the cell to hydroxylate
amino acids so that the skin can build peptides. Dietary C can be very
helpful, but there is clear evidence that topical C will increase activity
and collagen production in the skin. The problem comes when we
use so much vitamin C that we start inducing inflammation in the
skin. Usually less than 10 percent of unoxidized C is tolerated by most.
Those struggling with sensitive skin may need 5 percent or less.

Q Does diet affect acne?

A Absolutely. But not necessarily the way you think. Eating a candy bar
is not likely to create a specific acne lesion. However, if your overall
diet contains a lot of sugars or processed foods, or it promotes stasis
in the colon that reduces bowel-movement regularity, then you are
creating an environment that fosters bacteria, suppresses immune
activity, and may even increase sebum production.

Q Is oxygen good for my skin?

A Only when provided by your body. The skin carefully regulates oxygen transport by always providing antioxidant "bodyguards" at the
ready. Oxygen is important in the dermis and epidermis, but it also
quickly becomes our main source of aging. For this reason, I do not

recommend adding oxygen in any form including benzoyl peroxide and hydrogen peroxide.

Q Is aloe good for my skin?

A Yes, but buyer beware. There are drastic differences between the quality of aloe products. Many products have "aloe" in huge letters but only offer a small percentage of aloe, mixed with all kinds of inflammatory ingredients. For burned or damaged skin, fresh aloe from a plant can heal the skin dramatically. Organic aloe (90 percent or more) can offer benefits close to the plant source. Anything else has most likely lost a tremendous amount of its healing value.

Q Does shaving make facial hair coarse?

A No. It can certainly feel more coarse when it is shorter, but the evidence suggests that shaving will not cause a hair to go from being small, light-colored, and thin to thick, dark, and coarse. However, hair can change with hormonal influences.

Q Can anything that makes wrinkles disappear in five minutes be good?

A Not really. I suppose you could argue that temporary plumping has a purpose and can be a nice effect for an evening out. Egg proteins are an example of a topical that tightens the skin but does not trigger inflammation. Most other plumpers work primarily by creating an inflammatory event in your skin that makes the lines appear diminished. This can be done with a variety of ingredients: glycolic acid and L-ascorbic acid are two commonly used options. If it works that fast, it is not a rejuvenating event in the skin. But if you still want to try it, don't spend too much on plumpers because they are not worth the money.

Q Should I avoid parabens?

A Yes. I know a lot of chemists and formulators are still on the pro-paraben bandwagon, arguing that it is most important to control bacteria in the product. While I agree with the premise, there are many antibacterial options that are not as toxic. Parabens have been found in breast tumors, which is always a concern. Don't get too caught up in scanning labels for parabens because there are many terms for toxic preservatives that manufacturers are using to fool you into thinking that the product is paraben-free and preserved in a healthy way. Phenoxyethanol is also not advised for similar reasons.

Q Is there a difference between fragrance and essential oils?

A Yes. Fragrances are routinely toxic, while essential oils usually have a neutral effect on the skin. Some essential oils are irritating, but some can provide health benefits. On labels you may see "fragrance: essential oils" or something similar. European regulations require that skincare manufacturers put the word "fragrance" next to essential-oil names.

Q What are the top 10 ingredients to avoid when buying skincare products?

A
1. Parabens
2. Chemical sunscreens
3. Propylene glycol
4. Retinoic acid
5. Glycolic acid
6. Benzoyl peroxide
7. Hydrogen peroxide
8. Phenoxyethanol
9. Artificial colors
10. Artificial fragrance

Q What can worsen the effects of sun exposure?

A Smoking, drinking, copious food intake, exfoliating, overcleansing, sun-enhancing oils, and the use of too much topical oil in general.

Q Is lactic acid bad?

A Not at doses of less than 5 percent. Lactic acid is the only alpha hydroxy acid that is recognized by the skin. Our muscles make it along with other cells, and it is frequently deposited in the skin. In fact, it is a natural moisturizing factor. Like so many ingredients, the best results come from small doses. When used daily at concentrations above 5 percent, it starts to burn the skin, triggers exfoliation, and promotes skin starvation just like glycolic acid.

Glossary

Entry	Definition
ablative lasers	A laser that causes skin to vaporize or evaporate.
acne	A common skin disease that manifests in inflamed pustules on the surface of the skin.
acrochorda	Skin tags.
actinic keratosis	Pre-cancerous lesions.
alpha hydroxy acid	A naturally occurring acid derived from sugar cane, milk, apples, citrus fruits, and grapes that is used to exfoliate the surface of the skin. Includes glycolic acid, lactic acid, malic acid, citric acid, and tartaric acid.
angiogenesis	The formation of new blood vessels.
antioxidant	A substance that inhibits oxidation by combating free radicals.
atrophy	The wasting away of a part of the body.
avobenzone	A UVA protector found in some sunscreens. Also known as butyl-methyoxydibenzoylmethane and Parsol 1789.
basal cell carcinoma	The most common skin cancer, which rarely metastasizes to other organs because it grows locally.

basal layer	The deepest layer of the epidermis.
benzoyl peroxide	An oxidizing chemical used to treat acne.
benzophenone	A common sunscreen ingredient. Variants include dioxybenzone and oxybenzone.
Botox	Botulinum toxin that stops the displacement of collagen by keeping the muscles from separating the thinned collagen matrix in the dermis.
candida	Parasitic fungi that resemble yeasts and occur most often in the mouth, vagina, and intestines.
capillary	The body's smallest type of blood vessel.
ceramides	A part of the lipid structure that creates the protective glue that keeps the epidermis functioning properly.
chemexfoliation	Application of a chemical solution to the skin to burn the top layers, resulting in reduced fine lines, mild scarring, acne, and hyperpigmentation. Also known as chemical peels.
cinnamates	Chemicals frequently used to absorb UVB rays. Includes cinoxate, ethylhexyl p-methoxycinnamate, octocrylene, octyl methoxycinnamate.
cofactors	A substance that acts with another substance to bring about certain effects.
collagen	A fibrous protein that makes up the skin.
comedogenic	Something that clogs pores.
corneocyte	The top barrier of the skin in the stratum corneum and a key reflector of UV damage.
cortisol	A naturally occurring steroid produced by the brain in response to inflammation. The body's cortisol levels elevate in response to stress.
CO_2 laser	A common but aggressive ablative laser that vaporizes the top layers of the skin but also reaches the deeper layers of the dermis.

dermabrasion	Removal of skin imperfections by rubbing or scraping.
dermatitis	Any inflammation of the skin.
dermis	Located below the epidermis, this layer is the source of our skin's nutrition and most immune/repair activity.
eczema	Skin inflammation that causes lesions that itch and/or ooze, resulting in scaling or hardening of the skin.
elastin	A protein similar to collagen found in elastic fibers.
emulsifier	A substance that binds together two ingredients that normally don't mix.
enzymes	Protein produced by cells.
epidermis	The epidermis is the outermost layer of our skin. It does not have its own blood supply; instead, it forms a protective barrier on the surface of the skin and relies on the dermis to supply nutrients effectively.
erbium lasers	A common type of ablative laser that causes much less heat damage than a CO_2 laser but does burn away the surface of the skin.
erythema	Redness in the skin caused by increased circulation in the capillaries.
exfoliation	Removal of the skin's surface layer.
exogenous ochronosis	A condition that is marked by a bluish-black permanent pigment stain in the dermis.
fibroblast	A cell that produces and secretes collagen.
free radical	A type of particle produced in the body naturally or introduced externally (i.e., via pollution) that can damage the DNA of skin cells.
glabella	The area located between the eyebrows.
glycol	A chemical compound containing two hydroxyl groups. Listed on ingredient labels as propylene glycol, ethylene glycol, and polyethylene glycol (PEG).

glycolic acid	An alpha hydroxy acid found in grapes and sugar beets that's used as an exfoliant.
glycosamino-glycans	Polysaccharides that make up connective tissues. Also known as GAGs.
growth factor	A substance in the body, such as a hormone or cytokine, that can regulates cellular processes and stimulates cellular growth, proliferation, and differentiation.
Harmonized Water	Water containing a specific energetic frequency designed to provide different health benefits.
hemangioma	A tumor that's often benign and appears to be purplish or reddish.
holistic approach	Treating the entire body and mind rather than just separately treating its parts.
hyaluronic acid	A substance in the skin that the body uses to make connective tissue.
hydroquinone	A bleaching agent that removes pigmentation from the skin.
hyper-pigmentation	Darkening of the skin or fingernails in response to increased melanin levels. Hyperpigmentation may result from sun damage, acne, or other inflammation.
hypo-pigmentation	The discontinuation of melanin production to cells in a specific area.
immuno-suppression	The interruption or cessation of the immune system's natural responses.
inflammation	An immune response to cellular damage that is marked by capillary dilatation, redness, heat, and swelling.
intense pulsed light	High-intensity light using multiple wavelengths at the same time to cause capillaries to collapse, thereby reducing redness.
keratin	Protein that forms the chemical basis of epidermal tissues.
keratinocytes	The bulk of the cells within the epidermis.

keratosis pilaris	Bumps in the openings of the sebaceous glands that often appear on the thighs and/or arms.
L-ascorbic acid	The active form of vitamin C.
LED device	A heat-generating device that benefits the skin by improving nutrient delivery through an increase in circulation. Also triggers wound healing and collagen production.
lipids	The primary structure of cell walls that holds the epidermis together.
liposomal retinaldehyde	An acne treatment containing the liposome phosphatidylcholine, which has been proven to clear acne by 70 percent.
liposome	A minute sphere made of varying materials that are designed to either make ingredients mix better in solution, or more commonly to enhance penetration through the epidermis.
macrophages	Immune cells that ingest foreign matter.
melanin	A black, dark brown, reddish-brown, or yellow skin pigment.
melanocyte	An epidermal cell that produces melanin.
melanoma	The most dangerous skin cancer because it is likely to metastasize.
melasma	A discoloration of the skin's pigment. Melasma occurs across gender and ethnicity, but it is especially common in pregnant women or women taking certain contraceptives or undergoing hormone replacement therapy.
menthyl anthranilate	A UVA protector found in some sunscreens.
metallo-proteinases	Enzymes using a metal in the catalytic mechanism.
microderm-abrasion	A procedure in which the stratum corneum is partially or completely scrubbed off using jets of aluminum oxide crystals, other fine particles, or a rough surface in order to treat sun damage, scarring, and hyperpigmentation.

PABA (para-aminobenzoic acid)	A common sunscreen ingredient.
parabens	Chemical preservatives that researchers have discovered in breast tumors. Listed on ingredient labels as methylparaben, propylparaben, and butylparaben.
peptide	Two amino acids together. Used to treat rough skin and diminish wrinkle depth and volume.
pH	The measurement of acidity and alkalinity levels.
photorejuvenation	Treatment using intense pulsed light to remove wrinkles resulting from sun damage.
psoriasis	A condition that manifests in redness, irritation, and scaling of the skin.
retinoic acid	A form of vitamin A that's used to treat acne.
rosacea	Redness of the skin in areas of the face, including cheeks, nose, forehead, chin, or eyelids.
salicylates	Chemicals frequently used to absorb UVB rays. Includes ethylhexyl salicylate, homosalate, octyl salicylate.
salicylic acid	An anti-acne treatment.
sebum	A fatty substance manufactured by the sebaceous glands that helps move toxins through the dermis and out to the epidermis, where they can be shed. Also protects the dermis from dust and debris that can settle and irritate the skin from the outside.
septae	Fibrous connective tissue.
silica	An element that softens the skin and strengthens its connective tissue.
skin remodeling	The process by which our body removes damaged skin cells and replaces them with normal, healthy ones.

sodium lauryl sulfate	An inflammation-producing cleansing agent that's commonly found in face washes and liquid soaps.
spironolactone	A diuretic included in combination treatments for acne.
squamous cell carcinoma	The second most common type of skin cancer. It is associated with chronic UVB exposure.
steroids	Often prescribed to control inflammation in patients suffering from dermatitis, psoriasis, and eczema.
stratum corneum	The outermost layer of the epidermis.
stratum granulosum	The layer of the epidermis above the stratum spinosum, or granular layer, where keratin proteins and waterproofing lipids are produced and organized.
stratum spinosum	The layer of the epidermis known as the "spinous" or "prickle-cell" layer that has cells that produce lipids which prevent evaporation. Also where the production of keratin begins.
subcutis	A layer of tissue located below the epidermis that stores stem cells, vitamins, minerals, and cellular components.
titanium dioxide	A naturally occurring mineral that provides broad-spectrum coverage against both UVA and UVB rays.
T-zone	The area of skin most prone to oiliness—the forehead, nose, and chin.
ultrasound device	A heat-generating device that benefits the skin by improving nutrient delivery through an increase in circulation.
UVA (Ultraviolet A)	Invisible light rays from the sun that penetrate the skin more deeply than UVB radiation.
UVB (Ultraviolet B)	Invisible light rays from the sun known as the "burning rays" that penetrate only the outermost parts of the skin.

vasoconstriction	The closing of the blood vessels to limit blood flow.
vasodilation	Widening or opening the blood vessels.
vitamin K	Causes clotting in blood vessels, thereby eliminating discoloration.
zinc finger technology	A type of gene therapy that allows topical treatments to work at the cellular level.
zinc oxide	A naturally occurring mineral that provides broad-spectrum coverage against both UVA and UVB rays.

Selected References

INTRODUCTION

National Cancer Institute. SEER Cancer Statistics Review, 1973–1998. Available at http://seer.cancer.gov/csr/1973_1998/. Accessed April 7, 2010.

Rogers HW, Weinstock MA, Harris AR, et al. Incidence estimate of nonmelanoma skin cancer in the United States. *Archives of Dermatology*. 2010;146(3):283-287, 2006.

National Rosacea Society. Rosacea Awareness Month to Highlight Growing Incidence of Widespread Disorder. http://www.rosacea.org/press/archive/20100204.php. Updated February 4, 2010. Accessed April 7, 2010.

Simpson CR, Newton J, Hippisley-Cox J, et al. Trends in the epidemiology and prescribing of medication for eczema in England. *JRSM*. 102:108-117, 2009.

Icen M, Crowson CS, McEvoy MT, et al. Trends in incidence of adult-onset psoriasis over three decades: a population-based study. *Journal of the American Academy of Dermatology*. 60(3):394-401.2009.

Seebacher C. Candida in dermatology. Mycoses. 42 Suppl 1:63-67, 1999.

Baldo A, Bezzola P, Curatolo S, et al. Efficacy of an alpha-hydroxy acid (AHA)-based cream, even in monotherapy, in patients with mild-moderate acne. *Giornale italiano di dermatologia e venereologia*.145(3):319-322. 2010.

SmartSkin care.com. Reducing skin wrinkles with tretinoin (Retin-A®, Renova). Available at: http://www.smartskincare.com/treatments/topical/tretin.html Accessed April 27, 2010.

CHAPTER 1

Howard DL. How aging affects the structure of our skin. Dermal Institute Web site. Available at: http://www.dermalinstitute.com/idi/newIDIhome/txtonly_NEW/aging.htm#. Published April 2003. Accessed May 11, 2010.

Lucas T, Waisman A, Ranjan R, et al. Differential roles of macrophages in diverse phases of skin repair. *J Immunol.* 2010;184(7):3964-3977.

Stücker M, Struk A, Altmeyer P, Herde M, Baumgärtl H, Lübbers DW. The cutaneous uptake of atmospheric oxygen contributes significantly to the oxygen supply of human dermis and epidermis. *J Physiol.* 2002;538(Pt 3):985-994.

CHAPTER 2

Evolution of Lash Enhancers. Available at: http://www.fda.gov/downloads/Drugs/GuidanceComplianceRegulatoryInformation/EnforcementActivitiesbyFDA/WarningLettersandNoticeofViolationLetterstoPharmaceuticalCompanies/UCM182629.pdf. Accessed May 26, 2010.

The US Food and Drug Administration History. Available at: http://www.fda.gov/AboutFDA/WhatWeDo/History/default.htm. Accessed May 26, 2010.

The US Food and Drug Administration 1938 Food, Drug, and Cosmetic Act. Available at: http://www.fda.gov/AboutFDA/WhatWeDo/History/Product Regulation/ ucm132818.htm. Accessed May 26, 2010.

Pillai S, Oresajo C, Hayward J. Ultraviolet radiation and skin aging: roles of reactive oxygen species, inflammation and protease activation, and strategies for prevention of inflammation-induced matrix degradation—a review. *International Journal of Cosmetic Science.* 27(1):17-34, 2005.

Querleux B, Baldeweck T, Diridollou S, et al. Skin from various ethnic origins and aging: an in vivo cross-sectional multimodality imaging study. *Skin Research and Technology.* 15(3):306-313, 2009.

Barnes MJ, Constable BJ, Kodicek E. Studies in vivo on the biosynthesis of collagen and elastin in ascorbic acid-deficient guinea pigs. *Biochemistry Journal.* 113(2):387-397, 1969.

Roe DF, Gibbins BL, Ladizinsky DA. Topical dissolved oxygen penetrates skin: model and method. *Journal of Surgical Research.* 159(1):e29-36, 2010.

Thiele JJ, Hsieh SN, Briviba K, et al. Protein oxidation in human stratum corneum: susceptibility of keratins to oxidation in vitro and presence of a keratin oxidation gradient in vivo. *Journal of Investigative Dermatology.* 113(3):335-339, 1999.

CHAPTER 3

National Rosacea Society. If you have rosacea, you're not alone. Available at: http://www.rosacea.org/patients/index.php. Accessed May 10, 2010.

Essig MG. Chemical peel. WebMD. Available at http://www.webmd.com/skin-beauty/chemical-peel#ty7432. Accessed May 10, 2010.

Bradford PT. Skin cancer in skin of color. *Dermatological Nursing.* 21(4):170-7, 206; quiz 178, 2009.

CHAPTER 4

Westerhof W, Kooyers TJ. Hydroquinone and its analogues in dermatology—a potential health risk. *Journal of Cosmetic Dermatology.* 4(2):55-59, 2005.

McGregor D. Hydroquinone: an evaluation of the human risks from its carcinogenic and mutagenic properties. *Critical Reviews in Toxicology.* 2007; 37(10):887-914, 2007.

Olumide YM, Akinkugbe AO, Altraide D, et al. Complications of chronic use of skin lightening cosmetics. *International Journal of Dermatology.* 47(4):344-353, 2008.

Oral Treatment with Corticosteroids. The British Association of Dermatologists. Available at http://www.bad.org.uk/site/850/Default.aspx. Accessed May 20, 2010.

Petersen LJ, Lyngholm AM, Arendt-Nielsen L. A novel model of inflammatory pain in human skin involving topical application of sodium lauryl sulfate. Inflamm Res. 2010 Apr 1. [Epub ahead of print] Accessed May 27, 2010.

Parabens. U.S. Food and Drug Administration. March 24, 2006; Updated October 31, 2007. Available at http://www.fda.gov/Cosmetics/ProductandIngredientSafety/SelectedCosmeticIngredients/ucm128042.htm. Accessed May 20, 2010.

Darbre PD, Aljarrah A, Miller WR, Coldham NG, Sauer MJ, Pope GS. Concentrations of parabens in human breast tumours. *Journal of Applied Toxicology.* 24(1):5-13, 2004.

CHAPTER 5

Howard DL. How aging affects the structure of our skin. Dermal Institute Web site. Accessed at: http://www.dermalinstitute.com/idi/newIDIhome/txtonly_NEW/aging.htm#. Published April 2003. Accessed May 11, 2010.

Free radical. Merriam-Webster Online Dictionary. 2010. Available at http://www.merriam-webster.com/dictionary/free radical. Accessed May 8, 2010.

Understanding free radicals and antioxidants. Health Check Systems Web site. Available at: http://www.healthchecksystems.com/antioxid.htm. Accessed May 8, 2010.

Masaki H. Role of antioxidants in the skin: antiaging effects. *Journal of Dermatological Science.* 58(2):85-90, 2010.

Wu HC, Chang DK. Peptide-mediated liposomal drug delivery system targeting tumor blood vessels in anticancer therapy. *Journal of Oncology.* May 2010 (in press).

Muehlberger T, Moresi JM, Schwarze H, Hristopoulos G, Laenger F, Wong L. The effect of topical tretinoin on tissue strength and skin components in a murine incisional wound model. *Journal of the American Academy of Dermatology.* 52(4):583-588, 2005.

CHAPTER 6

Wise RA. Addictive drugs and brain stimulation reward. *Annual Review of Neuroscience.* 19:319-40, 1996.

Boisnic S, Branchet-Gumila MC, Le Charpentier Y, et al. Repair of UVA-induced elastic fiber and collagen damage by 0.05% retinaldehyde cream in an ex vivo human skin model. *Dermatology.* 199 Suppl 1:43-48, 1999.

CHAPTER 7

Lappe JM, Travers-Gustafson D, Davies KM, et al. Vitamin D and calcium supplementation reduces cancer risk: results of a randomized trial. *American Journal of Clinical Nutrition.* 85(6):1586-1591, 2007.

Reid IR. The roles of calcium and vitamin D in the prevention of osteoporosis. Endocrinology & Metabolism Clinics of North America. 27:389-398, 1998.

Bennett MF, Robinson MK, Baron ED, et al. Skin immune systems and inflammation: protector of the skin or promoter of aging? *Journal of Investigative Dermatology: Symposium Proceedings.* 13(1):15-19, 2008.

Rogers HW, Weinstock MA, Harris AR, et al. Incidence estimate of nonmelanoma skin cancer in the United States, 2006. *Archives of Dermatology.* 146(3):283-387, 2010.

Ting W, Schultz K, Cac NN, et al. Tanning bed exposure increases the risk of malignant melanoma. *International Journal of Dermatology.* 46(12):1253-1257, 2007.

Greenlee RT, Murray T, Bolden S, Wingo PA. Cancer statistics, 2000. *CA Cancer Journal for Clinicians.* 50:7-33, 2000.

Kricker A, Armstrong BK, English DR, Heenan PJ. Does intermittent sun exposure cause basal cell carcinoma? A case-control study in Western Australia. *Int J Cancer.* 60:489-494, 1995.

Gallagher RP, Hill GB, Bajdik CD, et al. Sunlight exposure, pigmentary factors, and risk of nonmelanocytic skin cancer I. Basal cell carcinoma. *Archives of Dermatology*. 131:157-163, 1995.

Preston DS, Stern RS. Nonmelanoma cancers of the skin. *New England Journal of Medicine*. 327:1649-1662, 1992.

US Cancer Statistics Working Group. United States Cancer Statistics: 1999–2005 Incidence and Mortality Web-based Report. Atlanta (GA): Department of Health and Human Services, Centers for Disease Control and Prevention, and National Cancer Institute; 2009. Available at: http://www.cdc.gov/uscs.

National Cancer Institute. SEER Cancer Statistics Review, 1973–1998. Available at http://seer.cancer.gov/Publications/CSR1973_1998/melanoma.pdf.

Westerdahl J, Ingvar C, Mâsbäck A, et al. Sunscreen use and malignant melanoma. *International Journal of Cancer*. 87(1):145-150, 2000.

Autier P, Dore JF, Schifflers E, et al. Melanoma and use of sunscreens: An EORTC case control study in Germany, Belgium and France. *International Journal of Cancer*. 61:749–755, 1995.

Kunz PY, Fent K. Estrogenic activity of UV filter mixtures. *Toxicology and Applied Pharmacology*. 217(1):86-99, 2006.

Wolff MS, Engel SM, Berkowitz GS, et al. Prenatal phenol and phthalate exposures and birth outcomes. *Environmental Health Perspectives*. 116(8):1092-1097, 2008.

Waters AJ, Sandhu DR, Lowe G, Ferguson J. Photocontact allergy to PABA in sunscreens: the need for continued vigilance. *Contact Dermatitis*. 60(3):172-173, 2009.

Gulston M, Knowland J. Illumination of human keratinocytes in the presence of the sunscreen ingredient Padimate-O and through an SPF-15 sunscreen reduces direct photodamage to DNA but increases strand breaks. *Mutation Research*. 444(1):49-60, 1999.

Rodriguez E, Valbuena MC, Rey M, et al. Causal agents of photoallergic contact dermatitis diagnosed in the national institute of dermatology of Colombia. *Photodermatology, Photoimmunology & Photomedicine*. 22(4):189-192, 2006.

Klammer H, Schlecht C, Wuttke W, et al. Effects of a 5-day treatment with the UV-filter octyl-methoxycinnamate (OMC) on the function of the hypothalamo-pituitary-thyroid function in rats. *Toxicology*. 238(2-3):192-199, 2007.

Beeby A, Jones AE. The photophysical properties of menthyl anthranilate: a UV-A sunscreen. *Photochemistry & Photobiology*. 72(1):10-15, 2000.

Gilchrest BA. If it's not the hamburgers, it's the sunscreens. *Journal of Investigative Dermatology*. 123(1):xi-xii, 2004.

Choksi AN, Poonawalla T, Wilkerson MG. Nanoparticles: a closer look at their dermal effects. *Journal of Drugs in Dermatology*. 9(5):475-481, 2010.

Paris C. A blocked diketo form of avobenzone: photostability, photosensitizing properties and triplet quenching by a triazine-derived UVB-filter. *Photochem Photobiol*. 2009;85(1):178-184.

CHAPTER 8

Tadokoro T , Kobayashi N, Zmudzka B, Ito S, Wakamatsu K, Yamaguchi Y, Korossy K, Miller SA, Beer JZ, Hearing VJ. UV-induced DNA damage and melanin content in human skin differing in racial/ethnic origin. *FASEB Journal*. 17:1177-1179, 2003.

Jackson BA. Nonmelanoma skin cancer in persons of color. *Seminars in Cutaneous Medicine and Surgery*. 28(2):93-95, 2009.

Langley RGB, Burton E, Walsh N, Propperova I, Murray S. In vivo confocal scanning laser microscopy of benign lentigines: Comparison to conventional histology and in vivo characteristics of lentigo maligna. *Journal of the American Academy of Dermatology*. 55(1):88-97, 2006.

Allegue F, Fachal C, Pérez-Pérez L. Friction induced skin tags. *Dermatology Online Journal*. 14(3):18, 2008.

Hahler B. An overview of dermatological conditions commonly associated with the obese patient. *Ostomy Wound Manage*. 52(6):34-36,38,40 passim, 2006.

Gupta S, Aggarwal R, Gupta S, Arora SK. Human papillomavirus and skin tags: is there any association? *Indian Journal of Dermatology, Venereology and Leprology*. 74(3):222-225, 2008.

Dianzani C, Calvieri S, Pierangeli A, Imperi M, Bucci M, Degener AM. The detection of human papillomavirus DNA in skin tags. *British Journal of Dermatology*. 138(4):649-651, 1998.

Mammas I, Sourvinos G, Michael C, et al. High-risk human papilloma viruses (HPVs) were not detected in the benign skin lesions of a small number of children. *Acta Paediatrics*. 97(12):1669-1671, 2008.

Jacobson MK, Kim H, Coyle WR, et al. Effect of myristyl nicotinate on retinoic acid therapy for facial photodamage. *Experimental Dermatology*. 16(11):927-935, 2007.

Bisset DL, Oblong JE, Berge CA. Niacinamide: A B vitamin that improves aging facial skin appearance. *Dermatological Surgery*. (7 part 2):860-865, 2005.

Fivenson DP. The mechanisms of action of nicotinamide and zinc in inflammatory skin disease. *Cutis*. 77(1 Suppl):5-10, 2006.

Jacobson MK, Kim H, Coyle WR, et al. Effect of myristyl nicotinate on retinoic acid therapy for facial photodamage. *Experimental Dermatology*. 16(11):927-935, 2007.

Oblong JE, Bissett DL, Ritter JL, et al. Niacinamide stimulates collagen synthesis from human dermal fibroblasts and differentiation marker in normal human epidermal keatinocytes: potential of niacinamide to normalize aged skin cells to correct homeostatic balance. 59th Annual Meeting American Academy of Dermatology; Washington, DC, 2001.

Gehring W. Nicotinic acid/niacinamide and the skin. *Journal of Cosmetic Dermatology*. 3(2):88-93, 2004.

CHAPTER 9

Acne. Dermaxime Web site. http://www.dermaxime.com/acne-information.htm. Accessed May 19, 2010.

Jocoy S. Vaginal yeast infections. Available at http://health.med.umich.edu/health-content.cfm?xyzpdqabc=0&id=6&action=detail&AEProductID=hw_knowledge base&AEArticleID=hw61044. Last updated June 17, 2008. Accessed May 19, 2010.

US Food and Drug Administration. Isotretinoin (marketed as Accutane) Capsule Information. Available at http://www.fda.gov/Drugs/Drug Safety/ PostmarketDrugSafetyInformationforPatientsandProviders/ucm094305.htm. Last updated February 23, 2010. Accessed May 20, 2010.

O'Donnell J. Overview of existing research and information linking isotretinoin (accutane), depression, psychosis, and suicide. *American Journal of Therapeutics*. (10)2:148-159, 2003.

Scheinfeld N, Bangalore S. Facial edema induced by isotretinoin use: a case and a review of the side effects of isotretinoin. *Journal of Drugs in Dermatology*. (5)5:467-468, 2006.

US Food and Drug Administration. Drug Safety. Available at http://www.fda.gov/ downloads/Drugs/DrugSafety/ucm085812.pdf. (40-41). Accessed May 23, 2010.

Isotretinoin and intestinal damage. *Prescrire International*. 17(96):154-156, 2008.

Garcia-Bournissen F, Tsur L, Goldstein LH, et al. Fetal exposure to isotretinoin— an international problem. *Reproductive Toxicology*. 25(1):124-128, 2008.

Malvasi A, Tinelli A, Buia A, De Luca GF. Possible long-term teratogenic effect of isotretinoin in pregnancy. *European Review of Medical and Pharmacological Science*. 13(5):393-396, 2009.

Vienne MP, Ochando N, Borrel MT, Gall Y, Lauze C, Dupuy P. Retinaldehyde alleviates rosacea. *Dermatology*. 199 Suppl 1:53-56, 1999.

Index

A

Ablative lasers, 50
Accutane, 63, 72, 154, 187
Acne
  after age 30, 189
  causes of, xiv, 146–49
  definition of, 145
  diet and, 192
  menstruation and, 189
  redness around, 11
  sebum and, 144–45
  treatment of, 33, 45, 150–58, 172
Actinic keratosis, 113, 118, 132, 133
African-Americans, 55, 125–26, 168
Age spots, 132, 137, 164–66
Aging
  inflammation and, xviii, 125–26, 177–78
  laser treatment of, 48–49
  reducing effects of, 136–37, 167–70, 173
  reversing, 188–89
  signs and symptoms of, 128–33
Alcohol, 79, 142, 171

Aloe, 193
Alpha hydroxy acids, xii, xv–xvii, 59–61, 72
Amino acids, 92, 103
Antiaging lasers, 48–49
Antibiotics, 65, 72, 147–48, 152–53
Antioxidants, 80–83, 102–3, 128, 166–67
Arms, bumps on, 187
Ascorbyl palmitate, 31–32
Avobenzone, 115

B

Basal cell carcinoma, 112
Basal layer, 5, 7
Bathing, 35, 79–80
Benzophenone, 114
Benzoyl peroxide, 33, 152–53, 186
Beta-endorphins, 94, 95
Botox, 130, 169, 183–84

C

Caffeine, 16, 66, 72
Candida albicans, 147, 149, 153, 159, 171

Capillaries
   role of, 138
   visible ("broken"), 43–44, 45, 130–31,
      189–90
Carbohydrates, digestion of, 92–93
Caviar, 191
Ceramides, 15, 70, 72, 85, 103
Chemical peels (chemexfoliation),
   51–54, 154, 166, 187–88
Chewing, 91, 104
Cinnamates, 115
CO_2 lasers, 50
Collagen
   boosting production of, 179
   breakdown of, 84–85, 129
   as ingredient in skincare products, 191
UV radiation and, 109–10
   vitamin C and, 30–32
Colon, toxin buildup in, 148–50
Corneocytes, 7
Cortisol, 94, 95, 97

D

Dental decay, 99
Dermatitis, xix
Dermis
   anatomy of, 8–9
   oxygen and, 32–34
   thinning of, 26, 28–30
Diet. See also Nutrition
   acne and, 192
   effects of, 141–44
   food combining, 93–94, 99–100
   inflammation and, 94–96, 142
   traditional, 99
Western, 89–90, 99
Digestion, process of, 90–93

E

Eczema, 64
Elastin, 109–10, 129

Epidermis
   anatomy of, 3–8
   protecting, 78–80
Erbium lasers, 50
Essential oils, 194
Estrogen, 116–17, 134–35, 146
Ethylene glycol, 70, 72
Exfoliation
   as common treatment, xvii
   effects of, 13–14, 36, 77–78, 176, 182
   frequency of, 56, 136, 182
   for hyperpigmentation, 166
   natural cycle of, 76
Eyes, puffiness under, 186

F

Facial Infusion™, 54, 156–57
Fats, 99
Fiber, 143, 155
Fibroblasts, 8–9
Fillers, 184
Fish, 96
Food combining, 93–94, 99–100
Fragrances, 194
Free radicals, 22–23, 82, 110, 128

G

Glycolic acid, xii, xvi, xviii, 59–60, 72,
   185
Glycols, 70, 72
Glycosaminoglycans (GAGs), 8–9
Grains, whole vs. refined, 98

H

Hair
   facial, 189, 193
   follicles, 133–34, 144
Harmonized Water, 119, 120, 157, 161
Heat devices, 51
Helicobacter pylori, 159
Hemangiomas, 134

HPV (human papilloma virus), 135
Hyaluronic acid, 184
Hydration, 100
Hydrogen peroxide, 33–34
Hydroquinone, 63–64, 72, 190–91
Hyperpigmentation, 47–48, 63–64,
    131–33, 162–67, 172–73
Hypopigmentation, 131–32, 133

I

Immune system
    skin's role in, 128
    suppression of, 110–11
Inflammation
    aging and, 125–26, 177–78
    from food, 94–96, 142
    preventing, xxiv–xxv
    skincare treatments and, xi–xiii, xvii–
        xviii, 21–22, 31
    skin's response to, 10–12
Insulin, 95–96
IPL (intense pulsed light), 42
Isotretinoin. See Accutane

K

Keratinocytes, 4–5, 7, 111
Keratosis pilaris, 187

L

Lactic acid, 59–60, 194
L-ascorbic acid, 30, 66–68, 80, 102
Lasers
    ablative, 50
    antiaging, 48–49
    assessment of, 49, 51, 183
    definition of, 42
    pigment, 47–48
    popularity of, 41
    vascular, 42–47
LED therapy, 51, 154–55, 157
Lightening agents, 165

Lipids, 5, 103
Liposomal delivery, 67, 82, 100
Liver spots, 132, 189
Local eating, 98

M

Macrophages, 9
Malic acid, 59–60
Mandelic acid, 59–60
Melanin, 5, 24–25, 127–28, 137
Melanocytes, 5, 7, 111, 127, 164
Melanoma, 112
Melasma, 161–63, 172–73, 191
Menstruation, breaking out during, 189
Menthyl anthranilate, 115
Microdermabrasion, 54–56
Mineral makeup, 114, 185
Minerals, 98, 102
Moisturizers, 181–82
Moles, 134

N

Nanoparticles, 119
"Natural," definition of, 184
Niacinamide, liposomal, 138
Nutrition
    lack of, in food, 96–97
    skin health and, 25–27, 89, 104
    steps to optimal, 97–100
    topical, 80–83, 100–103, 104–5

O

Oils, 99
Organic food, 98
Organic skincare, 184
Oxybenzone, 114
Oxygen, 32–34, 71, 72, 153, 192–93

P

PABA (para-aminobenzoic acid), 114
Parabens, 69–70, 72, 193–94

Peptides, 14, 68–69, 72
Phytoestrogens, 135
Pigment lasers, 47–48
Polyethylene glycol (PEG), 70, 72
Pores, enlarged, 133–34
Progesterone, 134–35, 146
Propylene glycol, 70, 72
Psoriasis, xiv, xx, 64

R

Radio frequency devices, 51
Retin-A®, xxi, 13, 14–15, 63, 101
Retinaldehyde, 13, 61, 85, 100–101, 153, 157–58, 161
Retinoic acid, 13, 14–15, 28–29, 61–63, 72, 153, 181
Rosacea, xiv, 11, 46–47, 159–61, 172, 192

S

Salicylates, 115
Salicylic acid, 152–53
Scar tissue, 44–46, 151–52
Scrubs, 183
Sebum, 144–45
Shaving, 193
Skin
    adaptations by, 10–12
    aeration of, 188
    anatomy of, 3–10, 16–17
    defense mechanisms of, 127–28
    detoxification through, 171
    dry, 190, 192
    dull, 186
    functions of, 3, 16
    immunocompromised, 12
    interfering with, 12–16, 27
    moist, 182–83
    oily, 137, 192
    pH and, 151
    starvation of, 182
    tone, uneven, 131–33

Skin cancer, 111–12, 115–16
Skincare products. *See also individual ingredients*
    ingredients to avoid in, 194
    organic or natural, 184
    regulation of, 20
Skincare treatments. *See also individual treatments*
    history of, 19–21
    inflammation and, xi–xiii, xvii–xviii, 31
    long-term effects of, xv–xvii, 21–23, 56–57, 175–77
Skin conditions. *See also individual conditions*
    holistic approach to, xix, xxi–xxii
    increasing prevalence of, x
    inflammation and, xiii
    outmoded approaches to, x–xi
Skin health
    basics of, 75
    nutrition and, 25–27, 89, 104
    promoting, 85–87, 136–38, 178–79
Skin remodeling, xix, xx, 28
Skin tags, 134, 135
Slap test, 34
Smoking, 16
Soaps, 79–80
Sodium lauryl sulfate, 35, 69, 72, 79
SPF (sun-protection factor), 117–18, 185–86
Spider veins, 190
Squamous cell carcinoma, 112
SRGF-7 (Skin Repair Growth Factor 7), 118, 120, 121
Stem cells, 6
Steroids, 64–65, 72
Stratum corneum, 5
Stratum granulosum, 5
Stratum spinosum, 5
Stretch marks, 44–46
Subcutis, 10
Sugar, 95–96, 142, 156, 171

Sunburns, 11

Sun exposure. *See also* Sun protection
 benefits of, 15, 83–84, 120
 effects of, 109–11
 excess, 107
 factors worsening effects of, 194
 insufficient, 107
 intensity of, 187
 pain from, 190
 skin cancer and, 111–12

Sunlight, basics of, 108–9

Sun protection. *See also* SPF; Sunscreens
 determining need for, 181
 future of, 118–19
 options for, 113–14
 recommendations for, 119–20, 121

Sunscreens
 chemicals in, 113, 114–17
 efficacy of, 112
 history of, 20
 nanoparticles in, 119
 reducing use of, 120
 sunblocks vs., 113–14

Supplements
 amino acid, 92
 mineral, 98

Swelling, xv

T

Tattoo removal, 47–48

Testosterone, 134, 145, 146, 189

Toxins
 in the colon, 148–50
 storage of, 94, 97

Tretinoin, xxi

T-zone, 137, 151

U

Ultrasound devices, 51

UV radiation
 effects of, 109–11
 types of, 108–9

V

Vascular lasers, 42–47

Vasodilators, 138

Vitamins
 A, 61, 100–101
 B, 101
 C, 30–32, 66–68, 72, 80–81, 101–2, 166–67, 192
 D, 15, 83, 102, 107, 120, 121, 128, 177
 E, 102
 K, 66, 72

W

Washing, 35, 79–80

Wrinkles
 cause of, 111, 129–30, 169
 skin color and, 24
 temporary plumping and, 193

Y

Yeast, 146–47, 149, 153, 171

Z

Zinc
 finger technology, 118, 135, 163, 166, 179
 oxide, 119–20